A₂Zᵢₙ ER

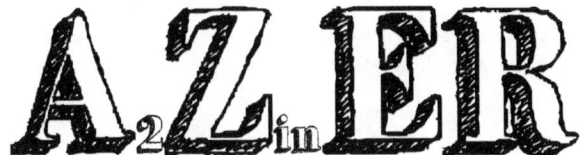

The Clinical Guide in the Emergency Room

Part 1
Diagnostics and Investigations

First edition
2019

Mina Azer
MSc., MBBCh.

Romany Azer
MD, MSc., MBBCh.

First edition: 2019

First Printing: May 2019

ISBN-13: 9781099150128

Imprint: Independently published

Mina Azer, MSc., MBBCh.
Specialist of general and visceral surgery.
Department of general surgery and emergency medicine, Ubbo-Emmius Klinik GmbH.
Oster Str. 110, 26506 Norden, Germany.
Email: meena_tharwat@yahoo.co.uk

Romany Azer, MD, MSc., MBBCh.
Specialist of anesthesia and intensive care.
Section of pain therapy,
Department of anesthesia, intensive care and pain therapy, Christliches Krankenhaus Quackenbrück GmbH
Danziger Str. 2, 49610 Quakenbrück, Germany.
Email: r.azer@ ckq-gmbh.de

Although every possible effort was made to ensure the accuracy of the information presented in this book, we cannot guarantee the absence of human error. It is also worth mentioning that we refuse to bear any moral or legal consequences by any means of false or incomplete management of patients based on information or knowledge acquired from this book. The medical field is an ever changing one, and it is the responsibility of the medical care provider to update their knowledge and skills, and to offer their patients the best possible management. One last fundamental point, medical treatment must be tailored to each individual patient. This unique management process should be the responsibility of the medical care provider along with the patient's informed consent without any predetermined management algorithms.

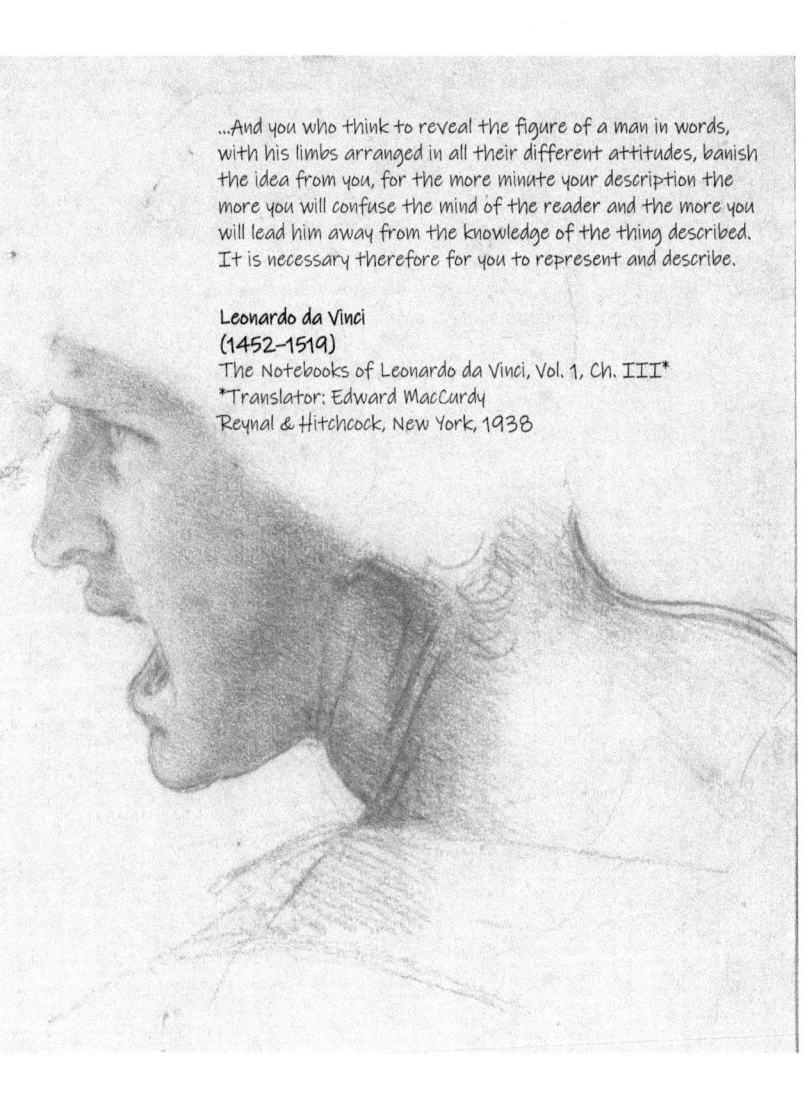

...And you who think to reveal the figure of a man in words, with his limbs arranged in all their different attitudes, banish the idea from you, for the more minute your description the more you will confuse the mind of the reader and the more you will lead him away from the knowledge of the thing described. It is necessary therefore for you to represent and describe.

Leonardo da Vinci
(1452–1519)
The Notebooks of Leonardo da Vinci, Vol. 1, Ch. III*
*Translator: Edward MacCurdy
Reynal & Hitchcock, New York, 1938

Acknowledgment

This work is inspired by my colleagues, both junior and senior. I was lucky enough throughout my career so far to encounter enthusiastic persons who were both eager to learn as well as pass their experience to others. This continuous process of sharing and learning was a main part of my work routine in the Gastroenterology surgical center in Mansoura University and The Egyptian Liver Institute.

I would also like to thank my colleagues in the surgery department in the Ubbo-Emmius Klinik in Norden, Germany, for being really supportive throughout the process of writing this book. I would like to thank Ibram Botros for his valuable insights and Samuel Gendy for his much appreciated technical support. Last but not least, I would like to thank Dr. Hripsime Rüstemyan and Dr. Hans-Uwe Volkers from whom I have learnt a great deal in the last three years.

This work could have never been done without the sincere support and understanding of my brave wife Mariam and my sweet angel Clara. I admit being an annoying person when consumed by a new idea. The good news is, I am done now!

Mina Azer

I would like to thank my parents, my lovely wife Annasimone Farid, my precious sweet children Sherry & John for their love, support and encouragement, and all my colleagues and mentors in Zagazig University in Egypt, Ubbo-Emmius Hospitals and Christliches Hospital Quackenbrück in Germany for their inspiration.

Romany Azer

TABLE OF CONTENTS

Chapter 1: General principles of radiological investigations   11

Checklist of ordering a radiological study   13
5 high yield suggestions by ARC regarding ordering radiological studies   15
Radiation safety   17

Chapter 2: Chest X-Ray   20

Normal Chest X-Ray   22
3 steps of Chest X-Ray evaluation   24

Chapter 3: Basic knowledge of computer tomography   27

Hounsfield units   30
Windowing   31
Projections   33
Contrast and phases   33
Interpretation, clues and tips   37

Chapter 4: Abdomen CT   39

Blood vessels   40
Liver   44
Kidneys and adrenal glands   51
Pancreas   52
Stomach and intestine   54
Spleen   55

Chapter 5: Brain and Skull CT   56

Blood   58
Cisterns   62
Brain   65
Ventricles   69
Bone   71
Conclusion   72

Chapter 6: Skeletal X-Ray   73

General concepts in evaluating skeletal X-Rays   74
Pelvis   76
Knee joint   80
Ankle joint   84
Foot   88
Shoulder joint   92
Elbow joint   96
Wrist joint and Hand   100
Lumbar vertebrae   104
Cervical vertebrae   108

Chapter 7: Emergency sonography (eFAST)   112

Introduction and basic concepts   113
Subxiphoid view   120
Inferior vena cava view   122
Right upper quadrant view   124
Left upper quadrant view   126
Pelvic sagittal view   128
Pelvic transversal view   130
Anterior thoracic view   132

Chapter 8: ECG   134

Introduction and basic concepts   135
ECG waves, segments and intervals   142
ECG changes with common cardiological conditions   150
Heart chambers hypertrophy or dilation   150
Myocardial ischemia   152
Myocardial infarction   154
Electrolyte disturbances   156
Heart block   157
Arrhythmia   159
How to write ECG report   163

Chapter 9: Laboratory tests   165

Arterial blood gases analysis   166
Complete blood count   174
Inflammation and sepsis parameters   176
Liver functions tests   178
Renal functions tests   180
Urine analysis   183
Coagulation profile   189
Pancreatic functions tests   192
Tumor markers   193
Cardiac profile tests   194
Summary and fishbone diagrams   195

PREFACE

This book is the first part of A₂ZᵢₙER© series which aims at providing a quick yet comprehensive source for medical care providers in emergency situations.

The beginning of the first night shift ever, is always a scary moment for everyone. The more experienced colleagues are already at home, and probably asleep. You are sitting in the ER or the ED waiting for the next patient, asking yourself, what would it be? A 2 cm cut wound or a perforated appendix? A mild gastroenteritis after an unfortunate fast food meal or a massive myocardial infarction? Knowing that all the possibilities are already lurking in the night outside, makes you a little bit nervous.

A₂ZᵢₙER© is the guide of the junior resident during their lonely night shifts. We assume that you have a good grasp of the basic medical knowledge. So, we won't discuss any theoretical aspects, mechanisms of action, or any other boring topics. All clutter has been ripped down leaving the very core of the addressed topics, bearing in mind the old – but still true – idiom; "common is common". In this book, you will find only the most common answers to the most common questions asked by younger colleagues.

The main idea of these books is to give you a handy tool that I wish I had during my first shifts. A concise guide to what to do and how to do it when you have no one to ask and no time to go through commercials, blocked content and false web search results to find a simple answer.

A₂ZᵢₙER© consists of 3 parts.

Part 1: Diagnostics and Investigation
A practical approach to medical diagnostic in the context of emergency situations. When to order a diagnostic test? how to perform it? and how to interpret its results? Diagnostic tests include ECG, Chest X-ray, skeletal radiology, Abdomen CT, Brain CT, Laboratory diagnostics and emergency sonography (eFAST).

Part 2: Clinical Classifications and Scores
Gallery of common bone fractures, classification and management, commonly used scoring systems and scales with a focus on emergency situations, and its interpretation according to the most recent guidelines.

Part 3: Management of emergencies
A brief and to-the-point management plan for polytrauma, nontraumatic acute chest pain, acute abdomen, and cerebral stroke. Glossary of frequently used medications (pain management, antibiotics, fluid therapy, etc..). Emergency maneuvers such as resuscitation, chest decompression, wound management, etc...

My last words to you: know the night philosophy! These could be summarized in the following points:

- ✓ Your main aim in the ER is not to miss a catastrophe more than to diagnose a rare condition.

- ✓ Stay focused on the patient's main problem. Do not get lost in the sideways.

- ✓ Learn to prioritize your actions, deal first with the problem that most likely would kill or deeply harm the patient.

- ✓ Do not perform any maneuver (diagnostic or therapeutic) during the night shift that could be postponed to the normal working hours in the next morning without harming your patient.

At last, my best wishes to my colleagues all over the world holding their position at night, guarding the human frontier against pain, suffering and death.

Mina Azer

Norden, 06ᵗ April 2019

CHAPTER 1

GENERAL PRINCIPLES OF RADIOLOGICAL INVESTIGATIONS

Contents

Checklist of ordering a radiological study   13

5 high yield suggestions by ARC regarding ordering radiological studies   15

Radiation safety   17

INTRODUCTION

It all began on 22 December 1895. Just 3 days before Christmas Wilhelm Roentgen, a German physicist, took the first photograph of a part of the human body using the newly discovered technique of X-Ray. This was a photo of his wife's Hand, who didn't forget to wear her ring for the photo session. Thus, the photo is still known as "Hand mit Ringen" or "Hand with rings". Roentgen presented this photo alongside his research results "On a new kind of ray: A preliminary communication" on December 28, 1895 to Würzburg's Physical-Medical Society journal. Since then, a new era of medical diagnostics took off.

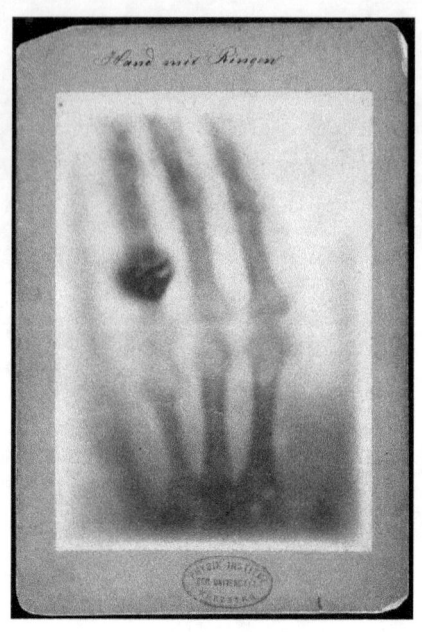

CHECKLIST FOR ORDERING A RADIOLOGICAL STUDY

Indication	✓ What is the diagnosis to be confirmed? ✓ What are the diagnoses to be excluded? ✓ What are the therapeutic consequences depending on the results of this study? If you failed to answer the above questions, do not perform the study!
Timing	✓ Are the above-mentioned diagnoses life threatening? ✓ Are the above-mentioned therapeutic consequences urgent? If the answer is yes, inform the radiology team to skip any waiting list for your patient. If the answer is no, perform the study with normal waiting time, allow time for other urgent patients and at least do not perform the study in the middle of the night!

Process	✓ What exactly is the ordered study?
	  o Patient ID (name, date of birth)
	  o Type (X-ray, CT, MRI, etc.)
	  o Site (head, thorax, ankle joint, etc.)
	  o Side when applicable (right or left)
	  o Views/projections (anteroposterior, posteroanterior, lateral view, etc.)
	  o Contrast type (iodine based, water, air, etc.)
	  o Contrast route (oral, per rectum, intravenous)
	  o Contrast phase in CT (triphasic, biphasic)

Precautions	✓ Is the patient pregnant, female in child bearing period or a child? If yes, consider alternative non-radiological methods when possible. ✓ Is the patient stable enough to undergo the study? ✓ Use of gonad shielding ✓ Use of safety measure (e.g. stiff neck with suspected cervical spine injury) ✓ For contrast studies: no history of contrast allergy ✓ For contrast studies: serum creatinine should be below 2 mg/dL.

A radiological study is only indicated when it adds a clear diagnostic value. You should have in mind a diagnosis to confirm or to exclude depending on the results of this study. Never order a study just to see what is going on!

Always remember to include the following in the written radiological study order:

- Patient confirmed ID
- Details of the process as described in checklist
- Urgency of the study
- Short description of the clinical picture
- Suspected diagnosis/differential diagnosis
- Precautions

FIVE HIGH YIELD SUGGESTIONS BY THE AMERICAN COLLEGE OF RADIOLOGY (ARC) REGARDING ORDERING RADIOLOGICAL STUDIES

These suggestions tackle the most common misconceptions regarding the use of radiological studies. Sticking to such suggestion could spare many patients unnecessary radiation exposure, time waste and stress. Also, its effect on resources sparing could not be overestimated.

1 Headache	**Do not do imaging study for uncomplicated headache** In the absence of specific risk factors for a structural disease as a cause of the uncomplicated headache, it is highly unlikely that the imaging study would add a value to the management process. Also avoid doing such studies minimize the chance of unnecessary procedures to clarify an incidental finding, which add nothing to the patients' well-being.
2 Pulmonary embolism	**Do not do imaging study to exclude pulmonary embolism in patient with low risk** In absence of clinical risk factors combined with a negative D-Dimer it is highly unlikely that CT-Thorax would add any new information.
3 Routine CXR	**Avoid admission or preoperative Chest X-ray for ambulatory patient with insignificant history and clinical examination** Chest X-ray should not be considered a part of the routine preoperative measures in minor or ambulatory surgeries.
4 Appendicitis in children	**Don't do CT Abdomen for children to evaluate a suspected acute appendicitis until after ultrasound has been considered as an option** Ultrasound in experienced hand is nearly as sensitive as CT in the evaluation of appendicitis in the pediatric population, but with the benefit of sparing the patient a load of radiation exposure.

	Don't recommend follow-up imaging for clinically inconsequential adnexal cysts
5 **Adnexal** **cysts**	Simple and hemorrhagic cysts in women during the child-bearing period are almost always physiologic. While in postmenopausal women small cysts are common and clinically insignificant. It is recommended to perform follow-up imaging only when the size of the cyst is more that the threshold value, which is 5 cm for women during the child-bearing period and 1 cm in postmenopausal women.

Other useful guide is The Appropriateness Criteria® (AC) of the ARC. These are evidence-based guidelines that describe the appropriate imaging study for each clinical condition[1].

---

[1] For more details visit the ACR website: https://www.acr.org/

RADIATION SAFETY

Although it revolutionized modern medical diagnostic methods, the introduction of X-ray came with a price. Exposure to such ionizing radiation can lead to direct harm (such as radiation burns), as well as damaging effects to the DNA (teratogenic or malignogenic effect). Such risks are magnified in certain groups of patients such as children, pregnant women and women in child-bearing period.

The risk depends on the amount of radiation passes through the soft tissues of the body. For example, CT uses by far more radiation than normal X-ray. Also, in X-ray of the abdomen, radiation passes through more tissue than in X-ray of the hand.

Last but not least, you should consider the cost of any investigation in terms of resources consumed (power, working hours of personnel and equipment) not to mention money paid by patients or insurance institution.

THE ALARA PRINCIPLE

ALARA is an acronym for "As Low As Reasonably Achievable." This is the key to balance the great benefit of radiological investigations with its risks and costs. It means: order radiological investigation "As Low As Reasonably Achievable" To reach a diagnosis.

> **ALARA principle**
> "as low as reasonably achievable" means using as low radiation as possible to achieve a clear diagnostic purpose. Simply, do not order radiological investigation unless it is clearly indicated.

If you clinically suspect a fracture of the fifth metacarpal bone, do not to hesitate to order a hand X-ray, because the very low risk of radiation exposure is not comparable to the risk of untreated fracture. But you don't need to X-ray the whole arm. Here, the exposure of upper- and lower arm in absence of clinical evidence of injury is more a tissue injury to the patient than a diagnostic maneuver. Remember the Hippocratic Oath! Do no harm!

In other words, use as low and few radiations possible to reach your diagnosis. But don't forget! You must reach your diagnosis.

RADIATION EXPOSURE

Because radiation can pass through the body, radiation dose is measured according to the amount of radiation received by the whole body. The scientific unit of measurement for whole body radiation dose, called "effective dose," is the millisievert (mSv). According to recent estimates, the average person in the U.S. receives an effective dose of about 3 mSv per year from natural radiation and cosmic radiation from outer space. This dose varies depending on your location. In Germany for example is about 2 mSv per year. This very low dose is nearly harmless. We receive more radiation doses throughout our life from none medical sources such as flying which according to the CDC leads to exposure of about 0.035 mSv of cosmic radiation in a flight within the United States from the east coast to the west coast. (approximately 6 hours- 11000 miles or 17700 km).[2]

To simplify the comparison between medical radiological exposure and the normal annual exposure to radiation, the following table state the amount of exposure of each type of X-ray or CT in terms of days of normal exposure as well as in mSv. One day of normal radiation exposure equals 0.008 mSv. So, the radiation exposure caused by the flight mentioned above equals approximately 4.5 days.

It is your burden to reassure a patient or terrified parent that the X-ray you just ordered won't hurt his/her son or daughter (using the table below). Or at least the very little possibility of risk is justified on the risk-benefit balance

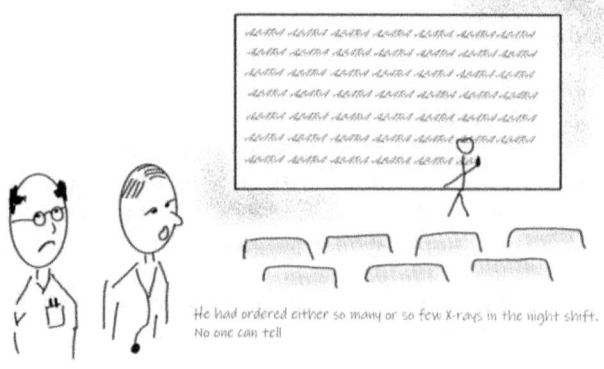

He had ordered either so many or so few X-rays in the night shift. No one can tell

[2] https://www.cdc.gov/nceh/radiation/air_travel.html

Procedure	Approximate effective radiation dose	Comparable to natural background radiation for:
Computed Tomography (CT)–Abdomen and Pelvis	10 mSv	3 years
Computed Tomography (CT)–Abdomen and Pelvis, repeated with and without contrast material	20 mSv	7 years
Computed Tomography (CT)–Colonography	6 mSv	2 years
Intravenous Pyelogram (IVP)	3 mSv	1 year
Barium Enema (Lower GI X-ray)	8 mSv	3 years
Upper GI Study with Barium	6 mSv	2 years
Spine X-ray	1.5 mSv	6 months
Extremity (hand, foot, etc.) X-ray	0.001 mSv	3 hours
Computed Tomography (CT)–Head	2 mSv	8 months
Computed Tomography (CT)–Head, repeated with and without contrast material	4 mSv	16 months
Computed Tomography (CT)–Spine	6 mSv	2 years
Computed Tomography (CT)–Chest	7 mSv	2 years
Computed Tomography (CT)–Lung Cancer Screening	1.5 mSv	6 months
Chest X-ray	0.1 mSv	10 days
Dental X-ray	0.005 mSv	1 day
Coronary Computed Tomography Angiography (CTA)	12 mSv	4 years
Positron Emission Tomography–Computed Tomography (PET/CT)	25 mSv	8 year

CHAPTER 2

CHEST X-RAY

Contents

Normal Chest X-Ray	22
3 steps of Chest X-Ray evaluation	24

INTRODUCTION

Chest X-Ray (CXR) is one of the most commonly used diagnostic tools in modern medical practice. In the following pages you will get a concise scheme of evaluating a CXR film through a simple 3-steps process. At first take look on the important anatomical landmarks of a normal CXR study. Go through the 3 steps as follows:

Step 1: confirm that you are examining the right study of the right patient at the right time. Also confirm the projection at which the film was taken. It could be either erect or bed study. Also differentiate between Anterioposterior study and posteroantenrior ones.

Step 2: evaluate the quality of the study to know to what extend could you rely on it to get a finding. For example, a malrotated study hinders good judgment of tracheal shift.

Step 3: spot the abnormality. Be sure not to oversee an important finding by going through the systematic ABCDE approach.

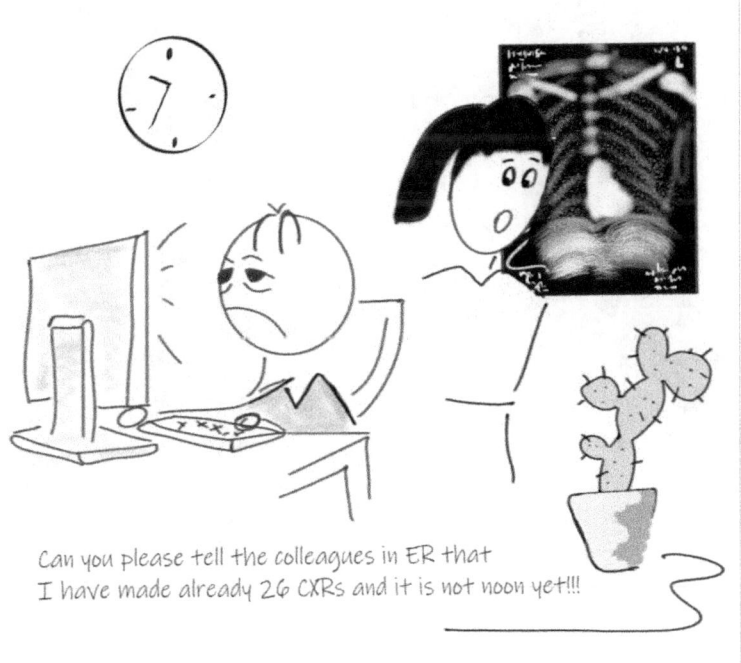

Can you please tell the colleagues in ER that
I have made already 26 CXRs and it is not noon yet!!!

Normal CXR

for more realistic view, compare the detailed picture below with the blank picture on the next page.

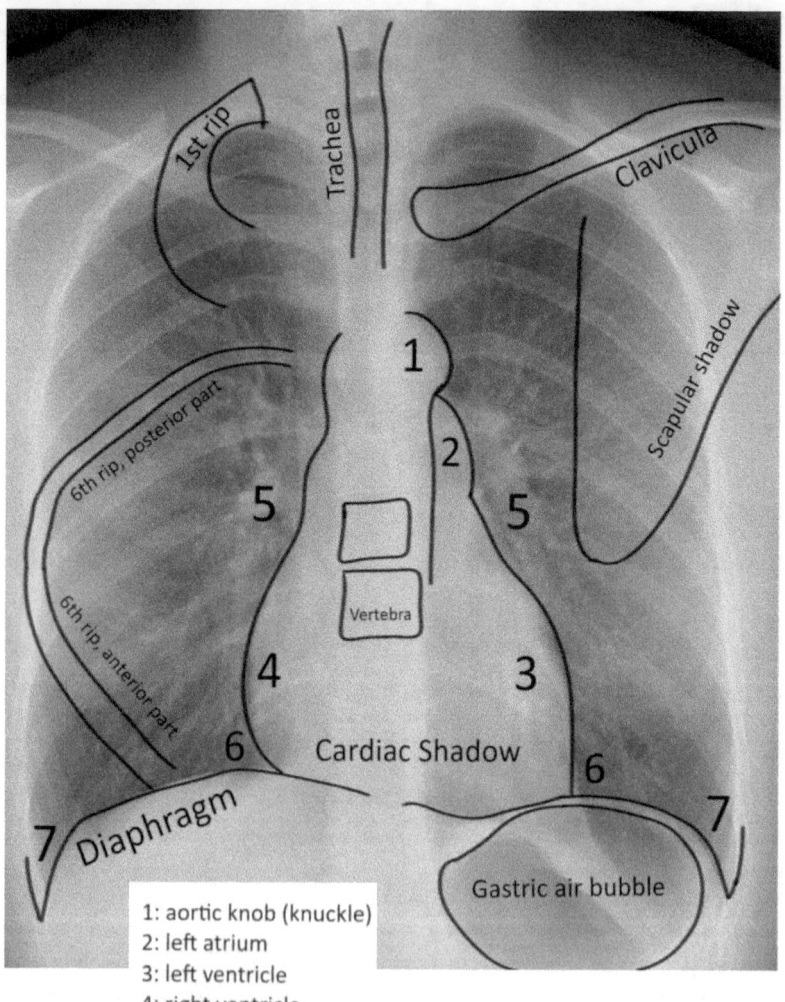

Vertebra

1

2

5

5

4

3

6

6

7

7

Cardiac Shadow

Diaphragm

Gastric air bubble

1st rip

Trachea

Clavicula

Scapular shadow

6th rip, posterior part

6th rip, anterior part

1: aortic knob (knuckle)
2: left atrium
3: left ventricle
4: right ventricle
5: lung hilum
6: cardiophrenic angles
7: costophrenic angles

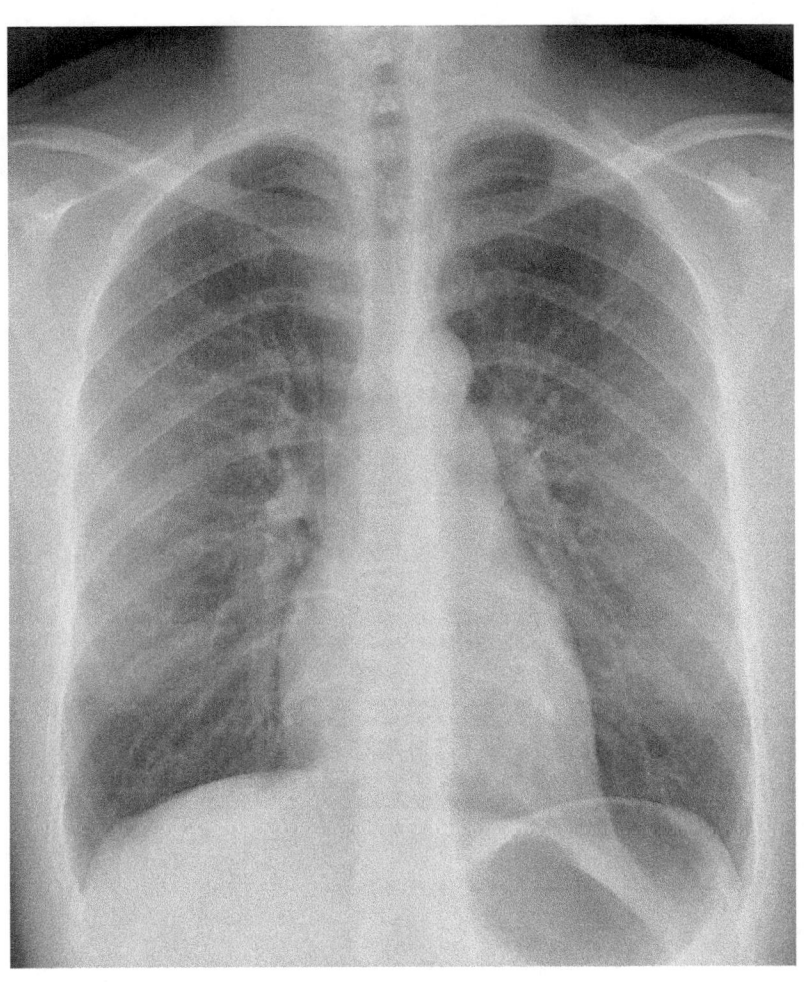

3 STEPS OF CXR EVALUATION

STEP 1: CONFIRM PATIENT AND FILM DETAILS;

Name, date of birth, date of the investigation

Projection: PA: Posterioanterior film: Erect/standing (standard) or AP: Anterioposterior film: laying (ICU or Polytrauma patients)

STEP 2: CONFIRM FILM QUALITY. (RIP)

Rotation	The 2 medial ends of the clavicle should be on the same distance of the spinous processes in between.
Inspiration	10th to 11th posterior rips should be visible in each lung field. Anterior 5th to 7th rips should intersect the diaphragm at the midclavicular line.
Penetration	The intervertebral spaces should be visible behind the cardiac shadow.

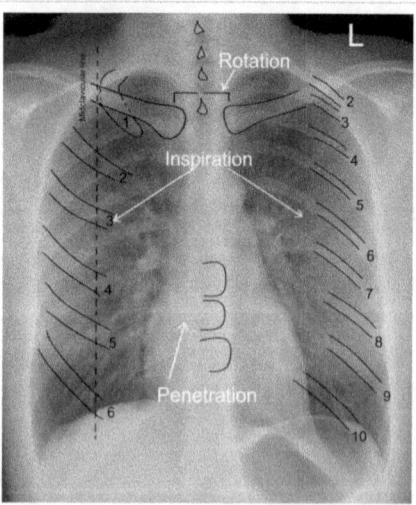

Inspiration vs Expiration

Chest X-Ray is usually done in full inspiration to accentuate the lung fields, except when pneumothorax is suspected where expiration film will accentuate the air in the pleural space.

STEP 3: SYSTEMATIC CHECK OF ABNORMAL FINDINGS (ABCDE SYSTEM)

Category	Normal finding	Abnormal finding
A: Airway	Trachea (darker air shadow) is central and the 2 main bronchi are visible	*Tracheal shift* • Towards the diseased side: Atelectasis, Pleural fibrosis and Pneumectomy. • Away of the diseased side: Pneumothorax, Pleural effusion and lung masses.
B: Breathing: Pleura, diaphragm and lung	Lung marking are visible bilaterally and fairly homogenous. Pleural angles (Costophrenic angels) are clear.	• Absent lung marking (Black shadow): Pneumothorax. • Absent of normal lung marking (White shadow): Atelectasis or effusion. • Inhomogeneous spots in lung field: Pneumonia (ill demarcated) or Tumor (well demarcated). • Obliterated Costophrenic angel: Effusion, blood or pus.

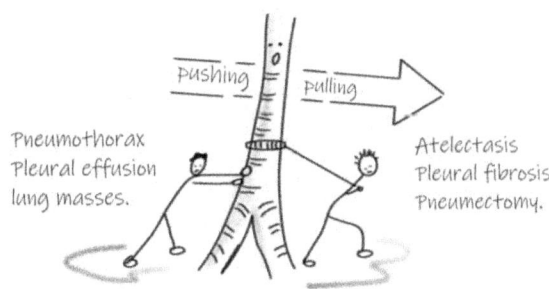

pushing   pulling

Pneumothorax
Pleural effusion
lung masses.

Atelectasis
Pleural fibrosis
Pneumectomy.

Tracheal shift
Tracheal shift can differentiate between 2 pathologies that appear at first identical (both are white shadow over the lung); Pleural effusion (pushes the trachea) and atelectasis (pulls the trachea).

C: Cardio	Anatomy of the cardiac shadow.	Larger cardiac shadow (more than 55%): Cardiomegaly.
	Normally the cardiac shadow is about 55% of the thoracic width	Flask shaped cardiac shadow is a sign of pericardial effusion.
D: Disability	Trace the borders of the clavicles and rips for fractures.	Irregularities in the borders of bones: Fracture.
E: Everything else	Instruments (Tracheal Tube, Pacemaker, Intravenous Port and Nasogastric tube) Gastric Bubble.	Air under the diaphragm is a sign of hollow organ perforation, while a gastric bubble is a normal finding in erect/standing X-ray.

Rips
Horizontal rips are posterior while oblique ribs are anterior.

CHAPTER 3

BASIC KNOWLEDGE OF COMPUTER TOMOGRAPHY

Contents

Hounsfield units	30
Windowing	31
Projections	33
Contrast and phases	33
Interpretation, clues and tips	37

CT is one of the powerful diagnostic tools that can be used in emergency as well as elective situations. But take care! it comes with a cost too.

- Radiation exposure
- Time delay in emergency cases
- Risk of allergic reaction up to anaphylactic shock due to i.v. contrast
- High cost

Indications of ordering a CT investigation are widely variable according to the site and the technique used. See figure on the next page.

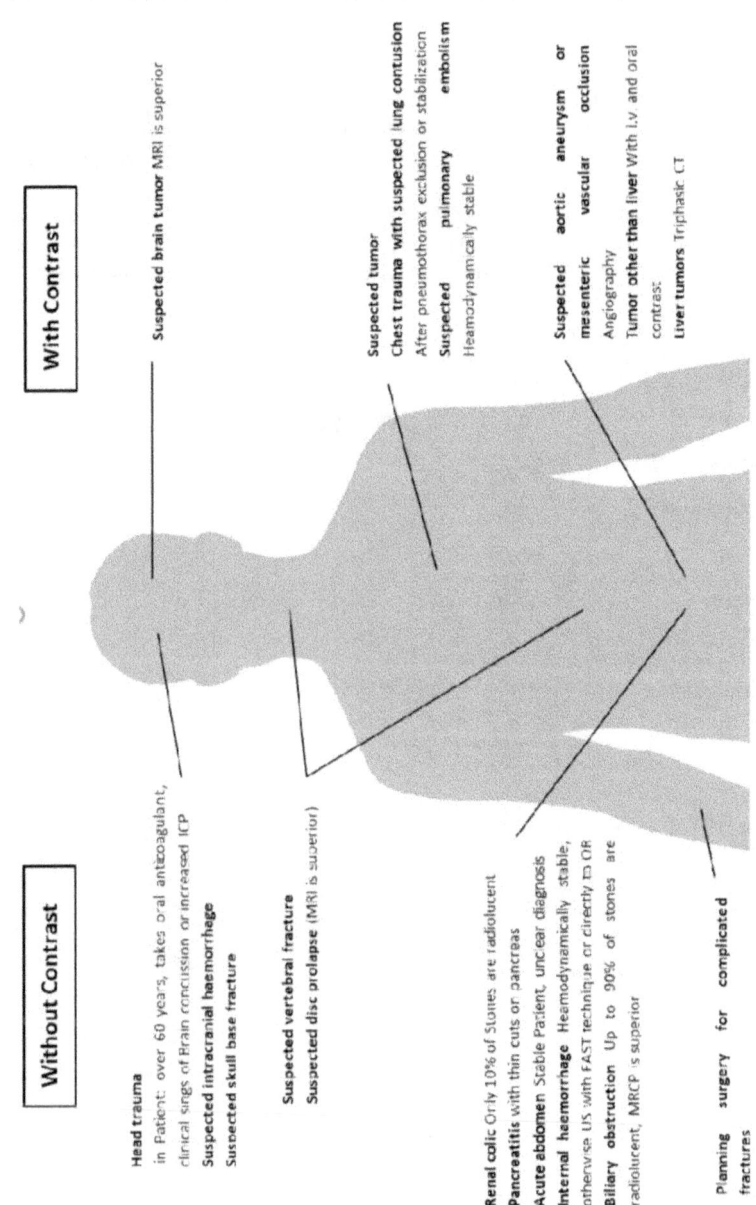

With Contrast

Suspected brain tumor MRI is superior

Suspected tumor
Chest trauma with suspected lung contusion
After pneumothorax exclusion or stabilization
Suspected pulmonary embolism
Heamodynamically stable

Suspected aortic aneurysm or mesenteric vascular occlusion Angiography
Tumor other than liver With i.v and oral contrast
Liver tumors Triphasic CT

Without Contrast

Head trauma
In Patient: over 60 years, takes oral anticoagulant, clinical sings of Brain concussion or increased IICP
Suspected intracranial haemorrhage
Suspected skull base fracture

Suspected vertebral fracture
Suspected disc prolapse (MRI is superior)

Renal colic Only 10% of Stones are radiolucent
Pancreatitis with thin cuts or pancreas
Acute abdomen Stable Patient, unclear diagnosis
Internal haemorrhage Heamodynamically stable, otherwise US with FAST technique or directly to OR
Biliary obstruction Up to 90% of stones are radiolucent, MRCP is superior

Planning surgery for complicated fractures

HOUNSFIELD UNITS (2000 SHADES OF GREY)

Structures are represented as shades of grey. The intensity (darkness or brightness) is measured in Hounsfield Units (HU or CT numbers). Each tissue has its own HU Value ranging from -1000 HU for air which appears Black to +1000 HU for dense bone or metal which appears bright white. The middle reference value is 0 HU, this represents pure water that appears grey.

The HU values of soft tissues are not universally standard. They may vary depending on a large spectrum of factors, including the manufacturer of the CT machine itself[3]. In the following table you can find the average values of some tissues rounded to an easy to remember figures.

Average HU values	
Bone	1000
Liver	60
White Matter	46
Grey Matter	43
Blood	40
Muscle	10-40
Kidney	30
Cerebrospinal Fluid	15
Water	0
Fat	-100
Air	-1000

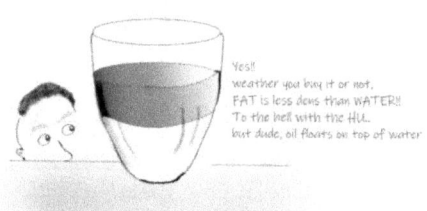

Yes!!
weather you buy it or not,
FAT is less dens than WATER!!
To the hell with the HU.
but dude, oil floats on top of water

Structure are described in relation to each other as Hypodens (darker), Isodens or Hyperdens (lighter).

[3] Lamba, R., McGahan, J. P., Corwin, M. T., Li, C.-S., Tran, T., Seibert, J. A., & Boone, J. M. (2014). CT Hounsfield Numbers of Soft Tissues on Unenhanced Abdominal CT Scans: Variability Between Two Different Manufacturers' MDCT Scanners. *AJR. American Journal of Roentgenology, 203*(5), 1013–1020. http://doi.org/10.2214/AJR.12.10037

WINDOWING

This means further processing of the image to accentuate a particular range of the HU scale. The human eye cannot recognize the slight difference of the grey shade. For example, the liver tissue has +60 HU value, water is 0 HU and fat is about -100. If we see this in a normal scale (2000 HU window) like the picture below, it will be hard to see the 3 types as separate structures. But if we want to examine this range closely, we better choose a soft tissue window. This means we make the computer only project tissues or values between +200 und -200 HU, ignoring other tissue like air or bone. Here +200 will be white, -200 will be black and values in between are shades of grey.

Other famous window is the bone window. Instead of projecting bone as a white homogenous spot, very dens parts will be white and less dens parts will be black. This is very useful in diagnosing bone fissures or a not dislocated fracture.

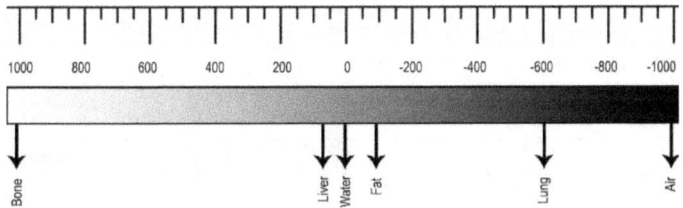

Each window is represented by 2 number:

- The window width (W): which describes the range of Hounsfield units displayed.
- The window level (L): this is the Hounsfield number in the center of the window width.

Common CT Windows	
Brain	W:80 L:40
Subdural Window	W:130-300 L:50-100
Stroke	W:8 L:32 or W:40 L:40
Soft tissues of head and neck	W:350–400 L:20–60
Lungs	W:1500 L: -600
Mediastinum	W:350 L:50
Abdomen soft tissues	W:400 L:50
Liver	W:150 L:30
Spine soft tissues	W:250 L:50
Spine bone	W:1800 L:400

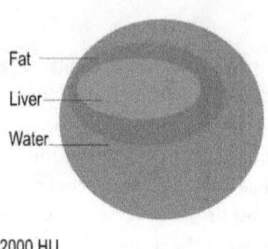

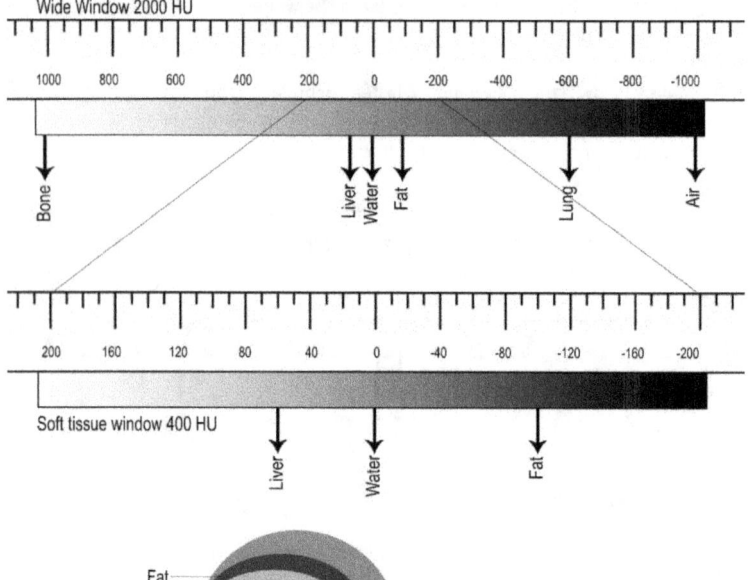

Wide Window 2000 HU

1000 800 600 400 200 0 -200 -400 -600 -800 -1000

Bone → Liver → Water → Fat → Lung → Air →

200 160 120 80 40 0 -40 -80 -120 -160 -200

Soft tissue window 400 HU

Liver → Water → Fat →

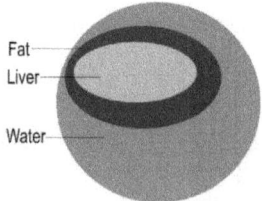

for example, this window has W: 400 and L: 0. This means the range
is 400 HU where the center is 0, i.e. +200 HU to -200 HU.

PROJECTIONS

there are 3 common projections in all CT scans (see the picture[4]):

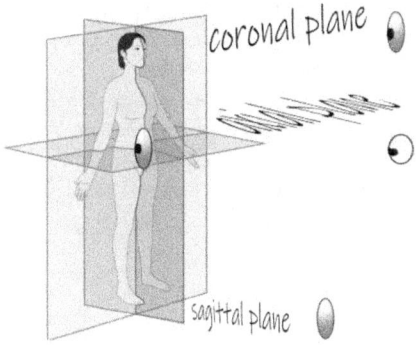

- Axial: the most familiar projection. Imagine that you are looking at the patient (sliced in the transverse plane) from downwards. The right side of the patient is also the right side of the picture.
- Sagittal: less commonly used.
- Coronal: similar to the projection of a normal X-ray.

CONTRAST AND PHASES

The aim of using a contrast in carrying out a CT Study is to enhance otherwise not clearly seen structures such hollow organs or blood vessels. Another benefit of using contrast is obtaining functional information about parenchymatous organs (eg. liver and brain) regarding its blood supply and venous drainage.

Using contrast in CT raise 3 main concerns

1. Allergy against iodine-based contrast that may lead to anaphylactic shock.
2. Nephrotoxicity of contrast (generally speaking the serum creatinine should be always less than 2 mg/dL before carrying out a contrast CT)
3. Increased radiation exposure. Each contrast phase doubles the overall radiation exposure of the examination.

---

[4] This picture was altered. Original source: OpenStax College. Anatomy & Physiology, Connexions Web site. http://cnx.org/content/col11496/1.6/

TYPES OF CONTRAST

- Oral contrast to enhance gastric and duodenal mucosa or anastomosis leakage.
  - Positive contrast: Barium or Gastrografin.
  - Negative contrast: Water.
- Contrast Enema to enhance rectal and colonic mucosa or anastomosis leakage.
  - Positive contrast: Barium enema.
  - Negative contrast: Air in virtual colonoscopy.
- Intravenous contrast to enhance blood vessels or parenchymatous organs according to the used phase.

PHASES

This term refers to the time interval between injecting the i.v. contrast and carrying out the CT scan. This time interval determines what blood vessels or organs in which the contrast reaches its highest concentration.

Phase	Timing after i.v. injection	Enhanced structures or tissues	Uses

Native or Non-enhanced CT	Before injection	none	• Baseline or reference to compare the contrast phases with.
			• Evaluation of Calefactions or fat such as in
			  o Calefactions or Stones (biliary or renal)
			  o Fat in tumors such as in adrenocortical adenomas
			  o Fat-stranding as seen in inflammation such as appendicitis, diverticulitis and omental infarction

Pulmonary arterial phase	6-13 sec	Pulmonary artery	Pulmonary embolism
Early systemic arterial phase	15-20 sec	Arteries, without enhancement of organs and other soft tissues.	Angiography
Arterial phase "late"	35-40 sec	All structures that get their blood supply from the arteries have optimal enhancement.	• Evaluation of blood supply • Hepatocellular carcinoma appears enhanced (supplied by hepatic artery)
Hepatic (most accurate) or late portal phase	70-80 sec	Liver parenchyma enhances through portal	Liver metastasis appears enhanced (supplied by portal vein).

		vein supply, normally with some enhancement of the hepatic veins.	
Nephrogenic phase	100 sec	All of the renal parenchyma enhances, including the medulla.	Detection of small renal cell carcinomas.
Systemic venous phase	180 sec	Systemic veins.	Detect venous thrombosis.
Delayed phase or "wash out phase"	5 to 15 min	Disappearance of contrast in all abdominal structures except for tissue with fibrosis	Fibrosis

Interpretation, Clues and Tips

The evaluation of any imaging study depends on good knowledge of the normal anatomy and how it looks like in this imaging study. In the next pages we will discuss the normal findings of 2 of the most commonly used CT studies; Abdomen CT und Brain CT. We will highlight also the most common pathological findings.

CT images is always evaluated as a series. Always use the scroll wheel of your mouse up and down to look at any particular structure. For the sake of simplicity, I will use the term of before and after to refer to superior and inferior structures respectively. When you start at the top of any given CT series, the superior structures will always appear *before* the inferior ones.

To evaluate CT images, you will need your 3D imagining skills. You will see 2D pictures on computer screen of 3D structures in the body. You must train your mind to go back and forth between 2D and 3D. The following examples could help.

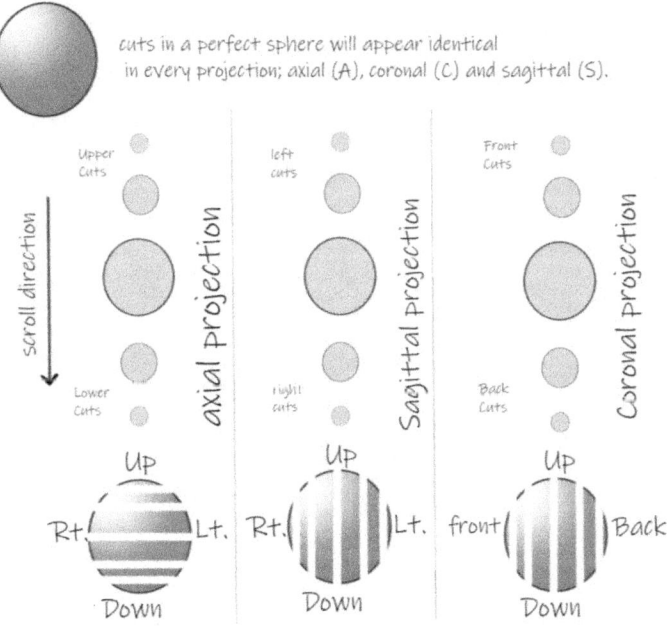

cuts in a perfect sphere will appear identical in every projection; axial (A), coronal (C) and sagittal (S).

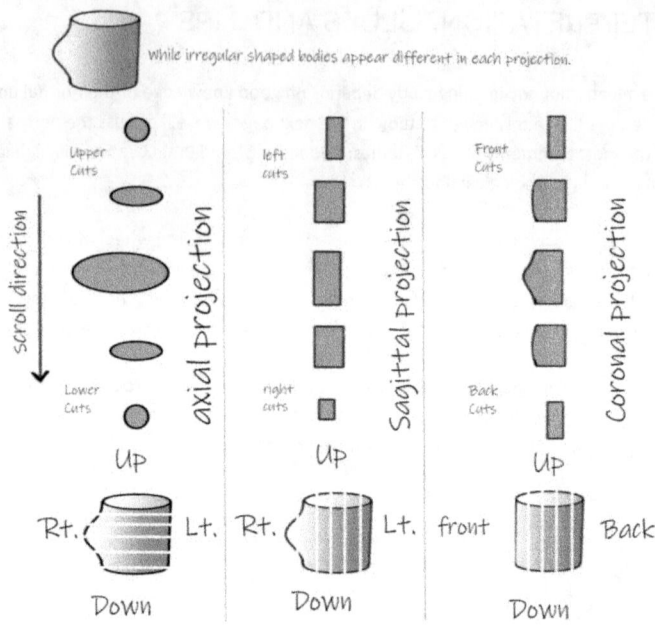

While irregular shaped bodies appear different in each projection.

Scroll direction

Upper Cuts

Lower Cuts

axial projection

Up

Rt. Lt.

Down

left cuts

right cuts

Sagittal projection

Up

Rt. Lt.

Down

Front Cuts

Back Cuts

Coronal projection

Up

front Back

Down

CHAPTER 4

ABDOMEN CT

Contents

Blood vessels	40
Liver	44
Kidneys and adrenal glands	51
Pancreas	52
Stomach and intestine	54
spleen	55

BLOOD VESSELS

Blood vessels in the abdomen are important landmarks that help you to navigate through different structures as they are usually easily recognized thanks to the intravenous contrast. They are glowing in an otherwise dark see of shades of grey. A good knowledge of blood vessels anatomy is vital in evaluating an abdomen CT. the easiest way to recognize these vessels is to start at the aorta to trace arteries as they originate or at the inferior vena cava (IVC) and portal vein to trace veins from there drainage backwards.

The coeliac trunk is the first to appear at the level of the first lumbar vertebra and soon divides into the common hepatic and the splenic artery.

coeliac trunk

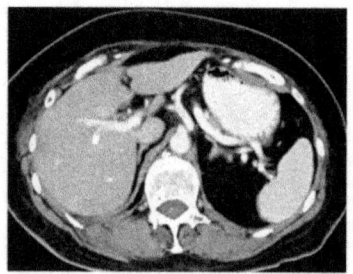

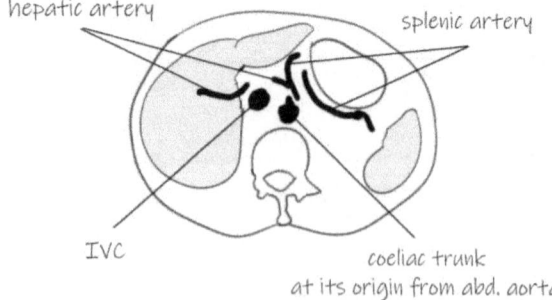

hepatic artery

splenic artery

IVC

coeliac trunk
at its origin from abd. aorta

The splenic artery could be traced along the upper border of the pancreas to the splenic hilum. It differs from the splenic vein by being tortuous.

Superior mesenteric artery arises from the aorta at the level of the first lumbar vertebra. This level is known also as the transpyloric plane. In this plan many other important features could be recognized.

- Pylorus stomach – hence the name.
- Left kidney
- Fundus of the gallbladder.
- Neck of pancreas.
- Superior mesenteric artery (SMA).
- Portal vein (PV).
- Left and right colic flexure.
- Spleen.

Transpyloric plan

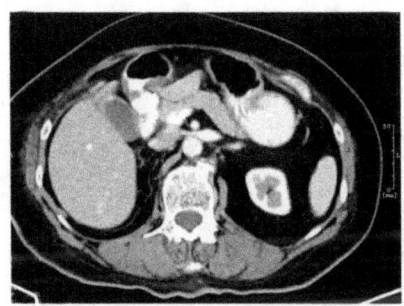

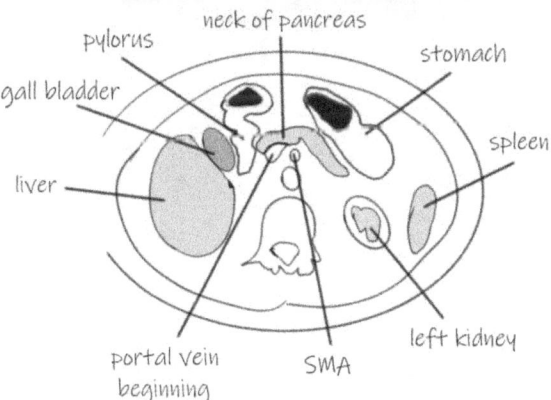

The renal arteries arise from the abdominal aorta at the level of the 2nd lumbar vertebra.

The inferior mesenteric artery arises from the abdominal aorta at the level of the 3nd lumbar vertebra.

The abdominal aorta ends at the level of the 4th lumbar vertebra by bifurcating into the common iliac arteries.

The portal vein with its tributaries and branches could be imagined as a *jumping gazelle* in the coronal view. *See the picture for details.*

Look for:

- **Mesenterial thrombosis:** discontinuation of the course of a vessel in CT with contrast or filling defect in contrast.

- **Aortic aneurysm:** dilatation of the diameter of the aorta more than 3 cm.

the portal vein

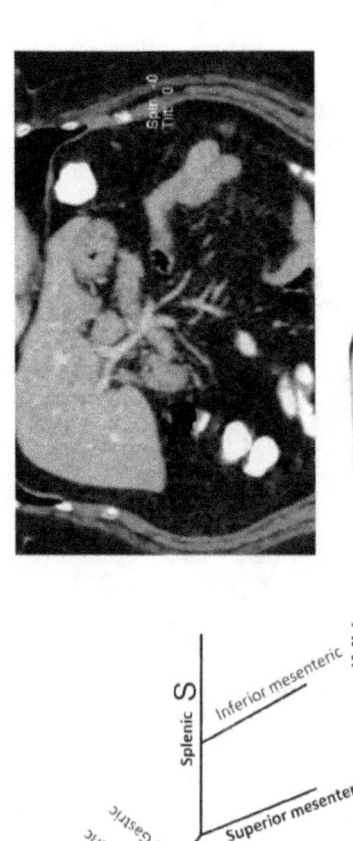

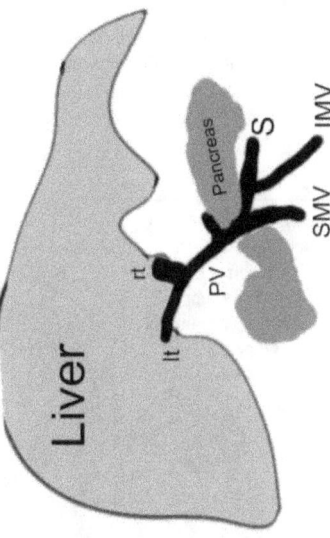

Liver

Pancreas

rt
lt
PV
S
SMV
IMV

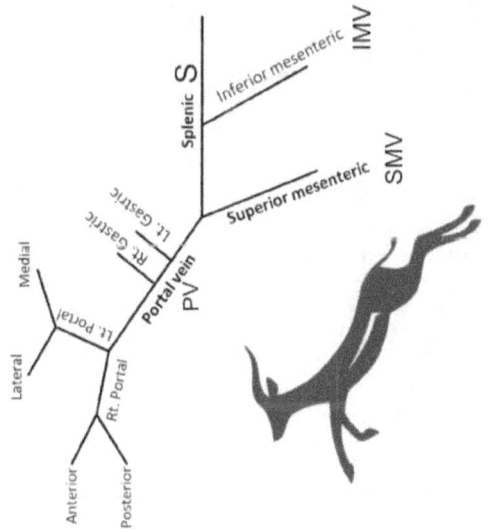

Lateral
Medial
Lt. Portal
Anterior
Posterior
Rt. Portal
Rt. Gastric
Lt. Gastric
Portal vein
PV
Splenic
S
Inferior mesenteric
IMV
Superior mesenteric
SMV

LIVER

Segmental anatomy of the liver is crucial to describe any abnormal finding. The definitive way to determine them is by relating them to the nearest hepatic and portal veins. As shown in the figure above the 3 hepatic veins divide the liver sagittaly into 4 sections. Each section is further divided transversally into upper and lower segment by the portal vein branch.

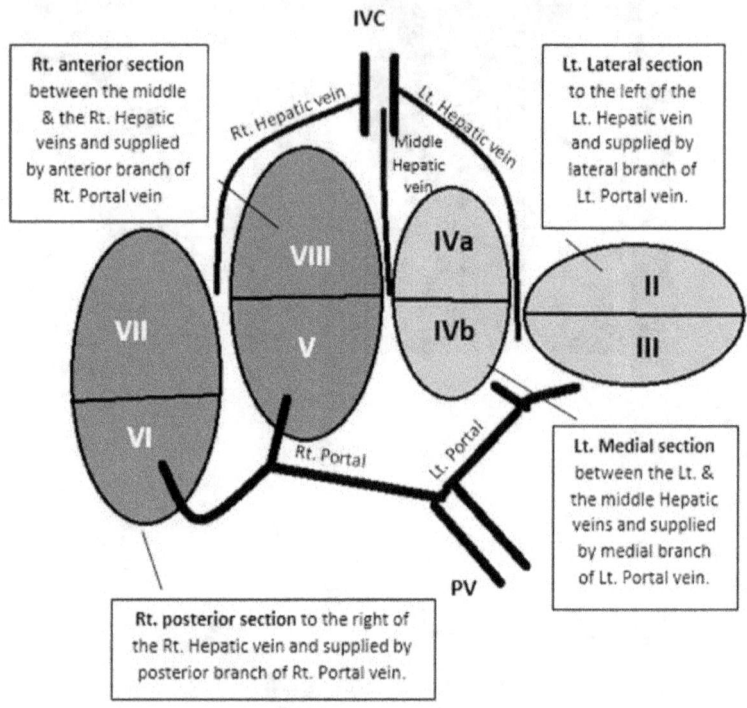

Hepatic upper segments

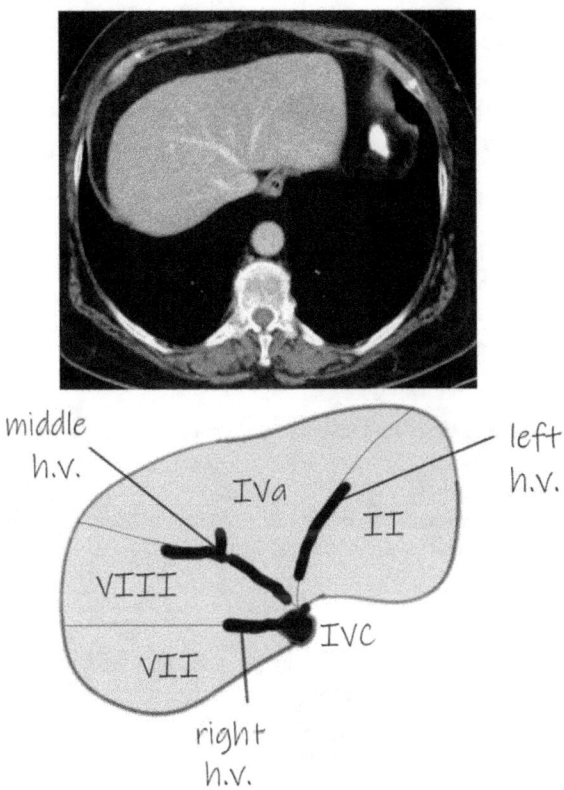

The left portal vein divides the left liver lobe into superior (II and IVa) and inferior (III and IVb) segments.

The right portal vein divides the right liver lobe into superior (VII and VIII) and Inferior (IV and V) segments.

Once the splenic vein appears, you can only see inferior liver segments (V, VI, IVb and III).

Sometimes it is a little bit tricky to demonstrate the hepatic veins. Here are tips to find the segments just by looking.

Liver Segments in order of appearance in axial CT cuts:

Segment VIII	The first to appear. The dome of the liver, appears with base of the heart in the same cut.
Segment II	Appears to the left from the falciform ligament before the left portal vein appears.
Segment IVa	Appears to the right from the falciform ligament before the left portal vein appears.
Segment I	Caudate lobe, just anterior and adjacent to IVC.
Segment III	Appears to the left from the falciform ligament after the left portal vein appears.
Segment IVb	Appears to the right from the falciform ligament after the left portal vein appears.
Segment VII	It is the far-right side of the liver as long as the IVC is seen impeded in the liver tissue.
Segment V	It is the gall bladder bed.
Segment VI	It is the far-right side of the liver. Begins as soon as the IVC leaves the liver tissue. The last to disappear.

first cuts to appear

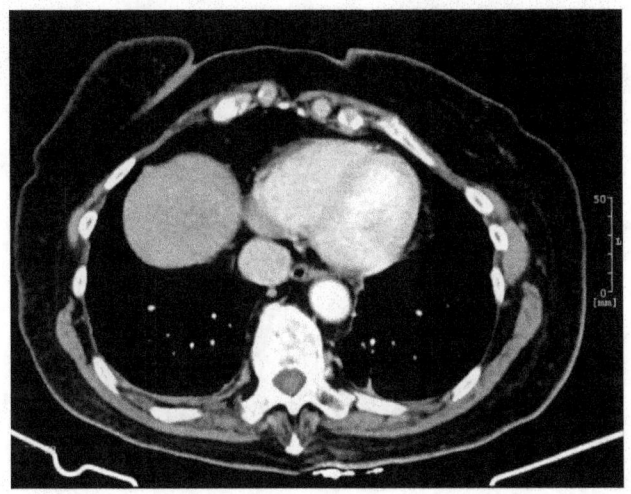

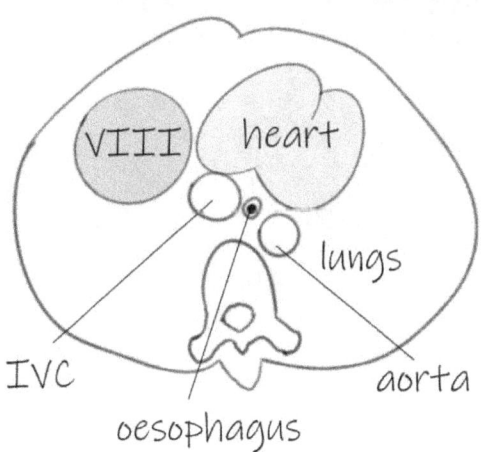

before portal vein appears

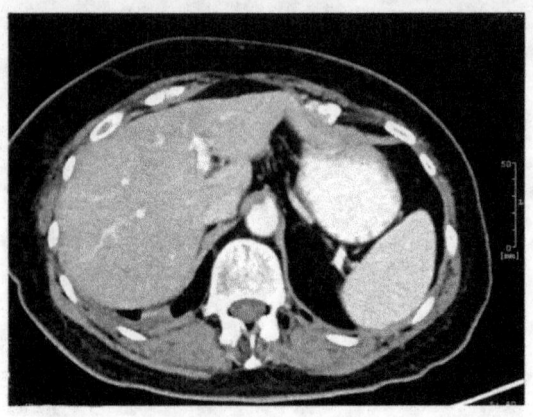

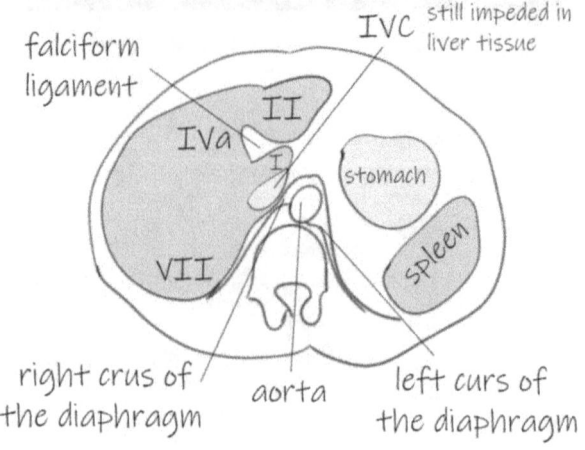

falciform ligament

IVa

II

I

VII

IVC   still impeded in liver tissue

stomach

spleen

right crus of the diaphragm

aorta

left curs of the diaphragm

after portal vein appears

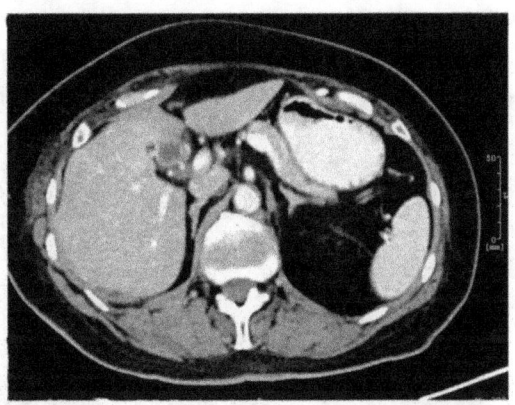

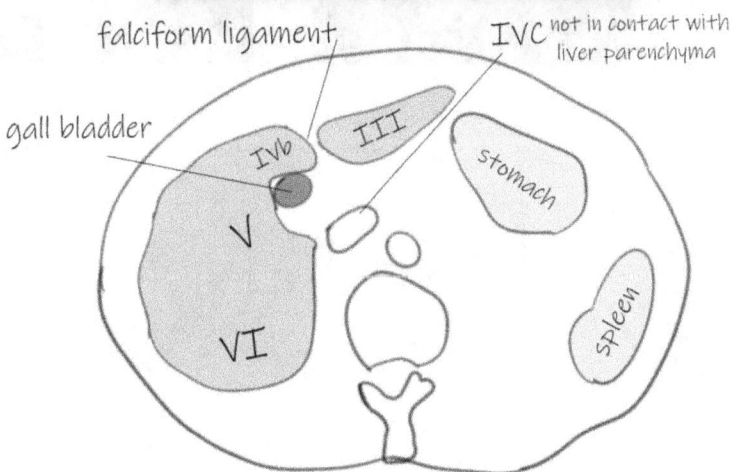

falciform ligament

gall bladder

IVb

III

V

VI

IVC not in contact with liver parenchyma

stomach

spleen

Look for:

- injury or hepatic lacerations
- Abscess with air-fluid level
- Hepatocellular carcinoma which looks brighter in arterial phase
- Metastatic lesions which looks brighter in portal phase
- Hemangioma which is identified by the closing iris sign, in which the contrast is washed away in the late washout phase from the center and outwards
- Dilated intrahepatic biliary radicles that indicated biliary obstruction.
- Gall bladder or common bile duct stones.

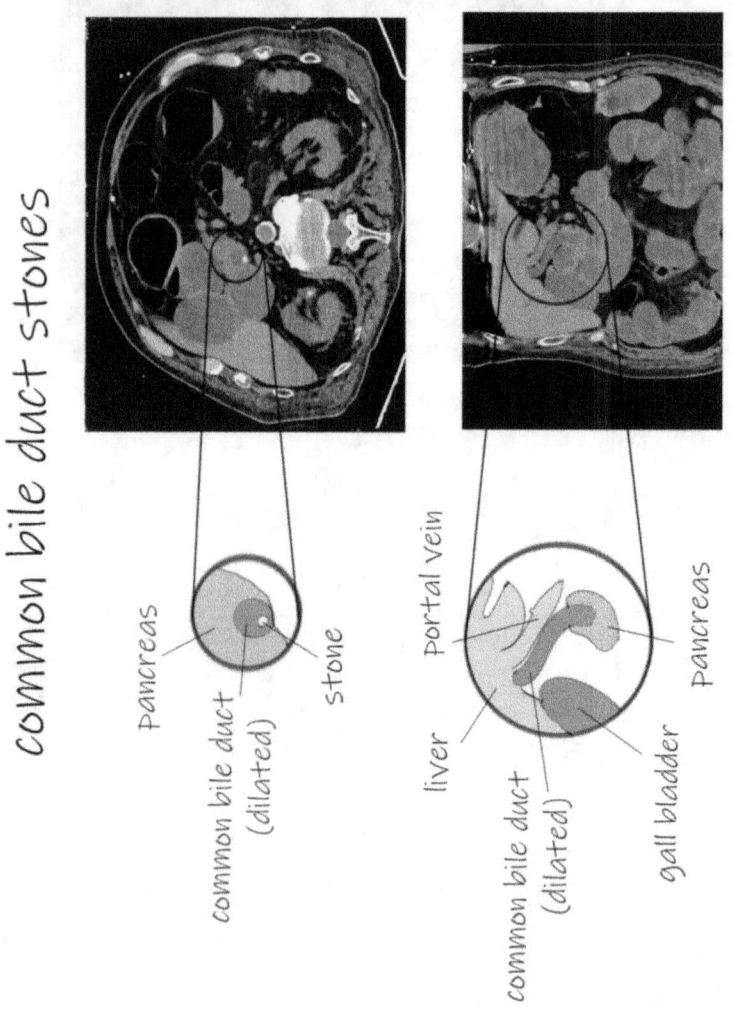

common bile duct stones

pancreas

common bile duct (dilated)

stone

liver

portal vein

common bile duct (dilated)

gall bladder

pancreas

KIDNEYS AND ADRENAL GLANDS

The kidney appears as oval-shaped organs on both sides of the vertebrae. The left kidney appears first as the right kidney is always pushed a couple centimeters by the liver. Renal cortex and medulla should be recognized with good differentiation specially in CT with i.v contrast. The ureter should be traced all the way down to the bladder to exclude stones, stenosis or dilatations. Renal arteries and veins should be easily traced to the Aorta or IVC respectively.

Adrenal gland appears as inverted Y-shaped structures the before the upper pole of the kidney appears.

Look for:

- Renal tumors
- Renal or ureteric stones. Look also for signs of back pressure (Hydronephrosis).
- Adrenal tumors, an accidentally found adrenal tumor without symptoms is called incidentaloma.

kidney and suprarenal

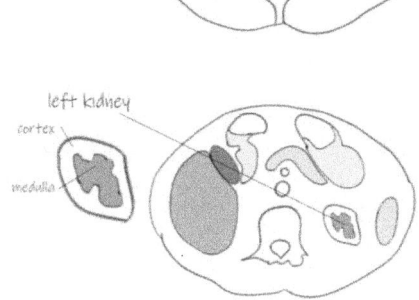
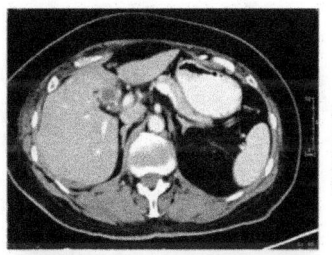
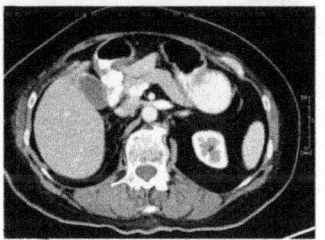

PANCREAS

The tail of the pancreas appears first at the hilum of the spleen due to the oblique position of the pancreas in the Abdomen. The body and the head can be traced in the lower cuts just posterior to the stomach. Another important landmark are the splenic vessels (see above). The confluence of the splenic vein and portal vein is the considered a landmark for pancreatic neck. Also, the superior mesenteric artery runs between the pancreatic neck and the uncinate process. This fact is used to determine the site of the uncinate process.

Look for:

- Pancreatic tumors. Always measure the diameter of the head of the pancreas. Greater than 3 cm diameter can be a manifestation of a pancreatic head mass. In this case the relation between the head (the mass) and the superior mesenteric artery is key to determine the resectability of the tumor.
- Acute pancreatitis could be manifested by diffuse pancreatic oedema and peripancreatic fluid.

> The lumbar vertebral body is about 3 cm in diameter. You can use it to roughly measure other structures.

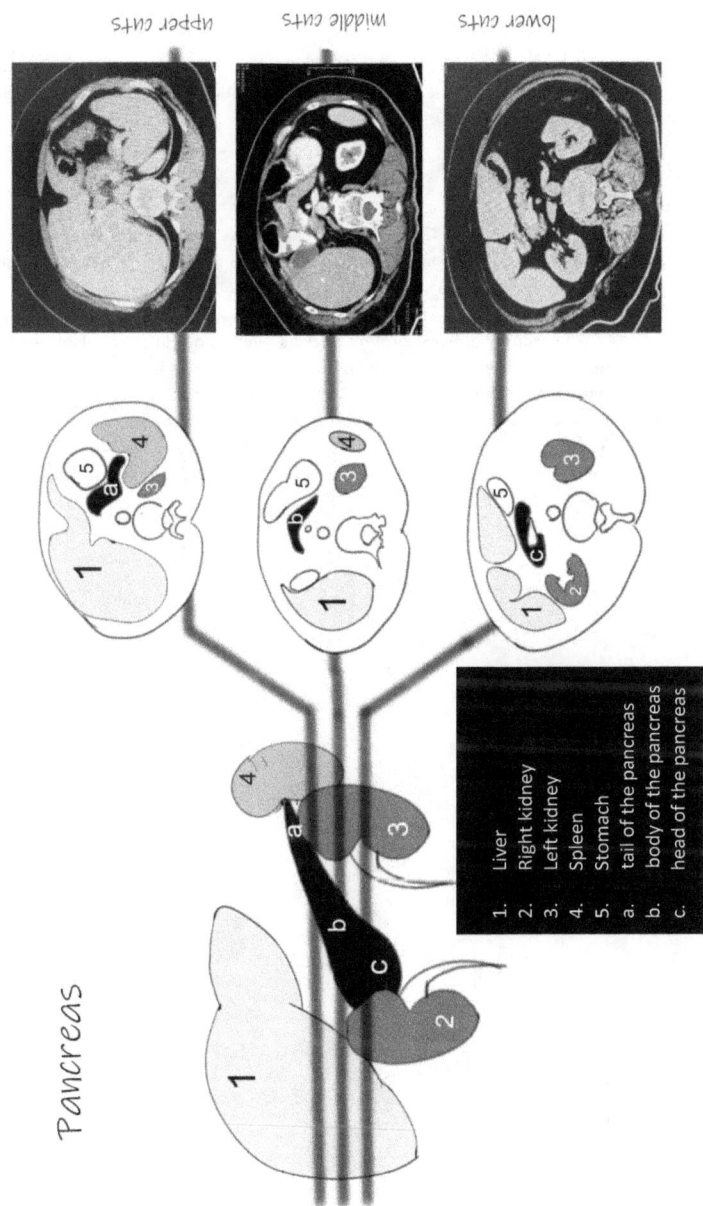

Pancreas

upper cuts

middle cuts

lower cuts

1. Liver
2. Right kidney
3. Left kidney
4. Spleen
5. Stomach
a. tail of the pancreas
b. body of the pancreas
c. head of the pancreas

STOMACH AND INTESTINE

It is hard to judge intestine as single loops. However, the overall view can give us important information. The large intestine is found on the edges, while the small intestine leis in the center.

Look for:

- Intestinal Obstruction: Caliber discrepancy of the small or large intestine especially in cases of mechanical intestinal obstruction due to adhesions, air-fluid level, obstructing lesion or incarcerated hernia.
- Mesenterial ischemia: visible defect or loss of continuity of a major blood vessel in CT with contrast or intramural air pockets, which is a sign of intestinal wall necrosis.
- Perforation: free air or extraintestinal gas.
- Diverticulitis: thickening of colon wall, visible diverticula or abscess.
- Appendicitis: oedema, wall thickening of appendix or periappendicular abscess.
- Gastric-outlet obstruction: dilated stomach usually due to fibrosed bulbar ulcer.
- Tumors: masses arising from the mucosa could only be seen with intraluminal contrast.

SPLEEN

Another parenchymatous organ in the abdomen that looks like a small liver on the left side. It appears just behind the stomach. Splenic artery and vein are usually easily recognized at the helium and should be traced back to the coeliac trunk and portal vein respectively. The splenic vessels are good markers for the pancreas, as they pass along its upper border (splenic artery) and posterior surface (splenic vein).

Look for:

- Signs of injury; splenic laceration or free fluid (blood).
- Areas of different texture that may indicate infarctions.

splenic injury

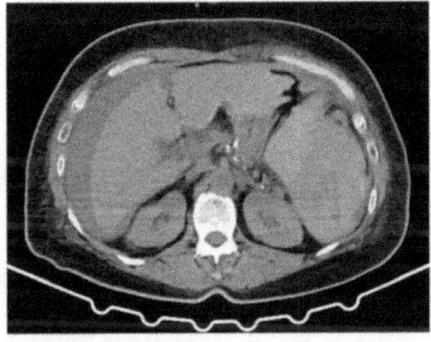

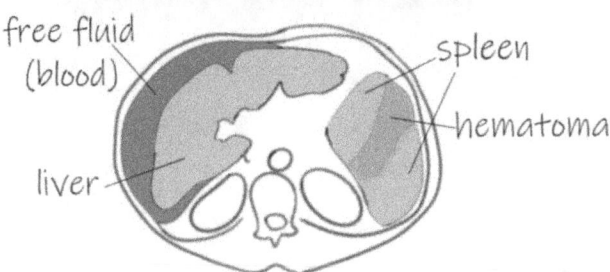

free fluid (blood)

liver

spleen

hematoma

> Calcification in arterial walls, simple cysts in liver or kidney are usually normal age-related findings.

CHAPTER 5

BRAIN AND SKULL CT

Contents

Blood	58
Cisterns	62
Brain	65
Ventricles	69
Bone	71
Conclusion	72

CT findings of brain and skull in emergency setting are divided into 2 broad categories:

1. Traumatic findings
   - Intercranial bleeding
   - Skull fractures
2. Stroke
   - Hemorrhagic stroke
   - Ischemic stroke

The following approach is meant for non-radiologists to be able to identify the 4 major findings as well as other important findings during the night shift. The main aim is not to miss a catastrophe.

Remember this Mnemonic: Blood can be very bad!

Blood	Can	Be	Very	Bad
Blood	Cisterns	Brain	Ventricles	Bone

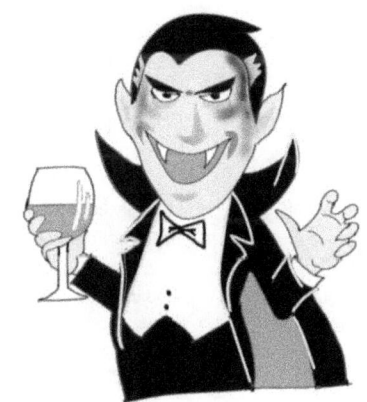

blood can NEVER be very bad!!

BLOOD

This means bleeding, either traumatic or due to rupture of aneurysm (hemorrhagic stroke). Acute bleeding (fresh clotted blood) in CT appears bright white or hyperdense, it turns Isodens at 1-2 weeks, while old hematomas (weeks or months old) appears darker or hypodense.

Normal finding: no extravascular blood. No bleeding.

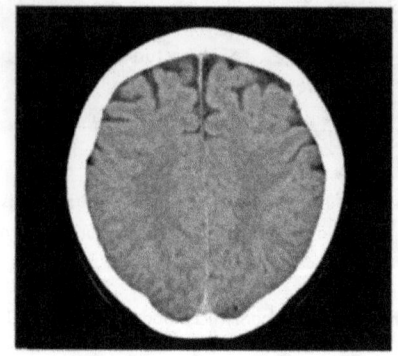

normal brain

	6 types of bleeding
Subgaleal hemorrhage	Extracranial hematoma of the scalp
Epidural hemorrhage	Lens-shaped, doesn't cross skull suture lines, can lead to midline shift or mass effect
Subdural hemorrhage	Sickle-shaped, crosses skull suture lines, can lead to midline shift or mass effect
Intraparenchymal hemorrhage	Especially in basal ganglia, ill-defined shape, can lead to midline shift or mass effect
Intraventricular hemorrhage	Blood in ventricles
Subarachnoid hemorrhage	Blood in cisterns

Epidural and Subgaleal hemorrhage

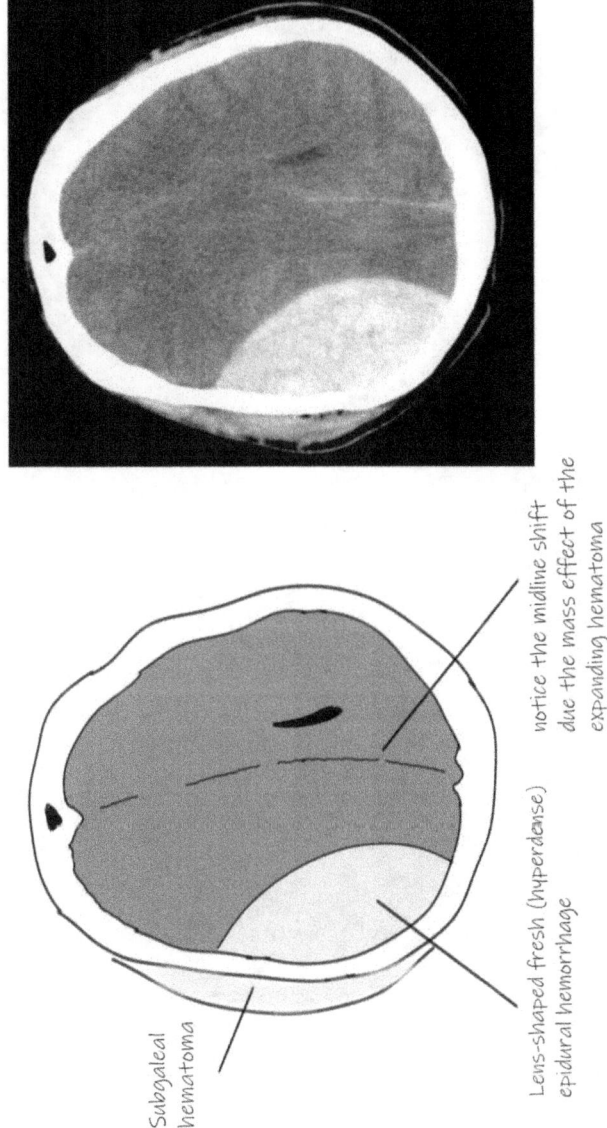

notice the midline shift due to the mass effect of the expanding hematoma

Lens-shaped fresh (hyperdense) epidural hemorrhage

Subgaleal hematoma

Subdural and Subgaleal hemorrhage

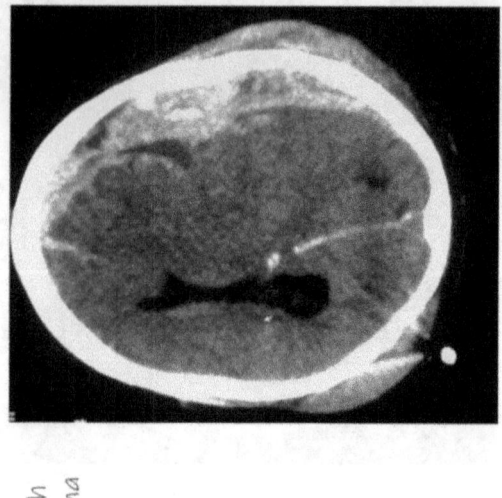

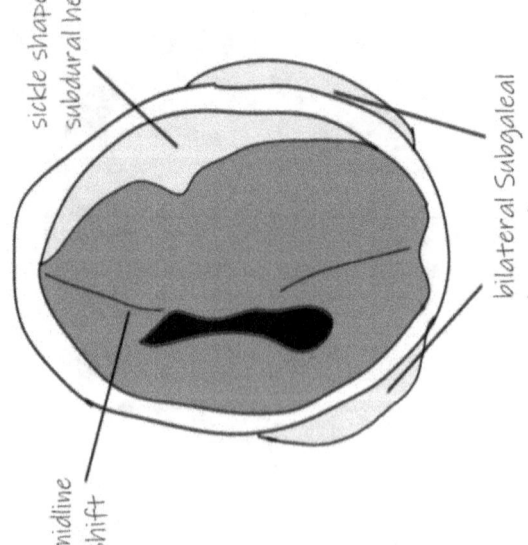

sickle shaped fresh
Subdural hematoma

bilateral Subgaleal
hemorrhage

midline
shift

Intraparenchymal hemorrhage

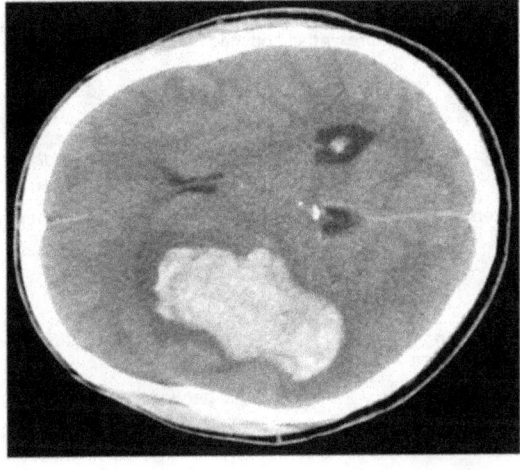

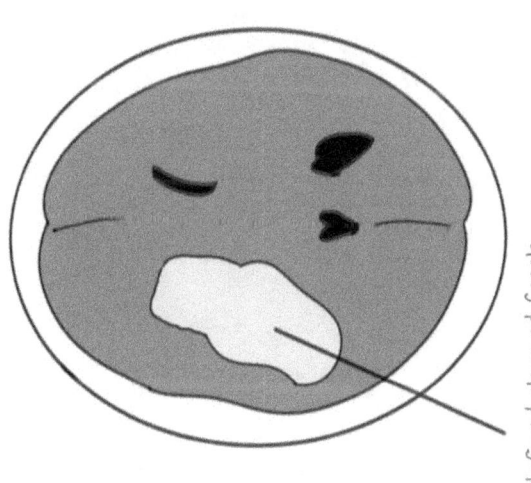

ill-defined shaped fresh
Intraparenchymal hemorrhage

CISTERNS

Cisterns are CSF collections coating the brain. They usually appear black or hypodense. Look for blood (white color) in cisterns which is a sign of subarachnoid hemorrhage.

Normal finding: All cisterns are present and opened (dark or hypodense)

4 important cisterns	
Circummesencephalic Cistern	Ring around midbrain (Ring coating a heart)
Suprasellar Cistern	Star-shaped just above midbrain, near circle of Willis and the pituitary gland (Sella Turcica)
Quadrigeminal Cistern	W-shaped, just anterior to the cerebellum
Sylvian Cistern	Y-shaped between frontal and temporal lobe

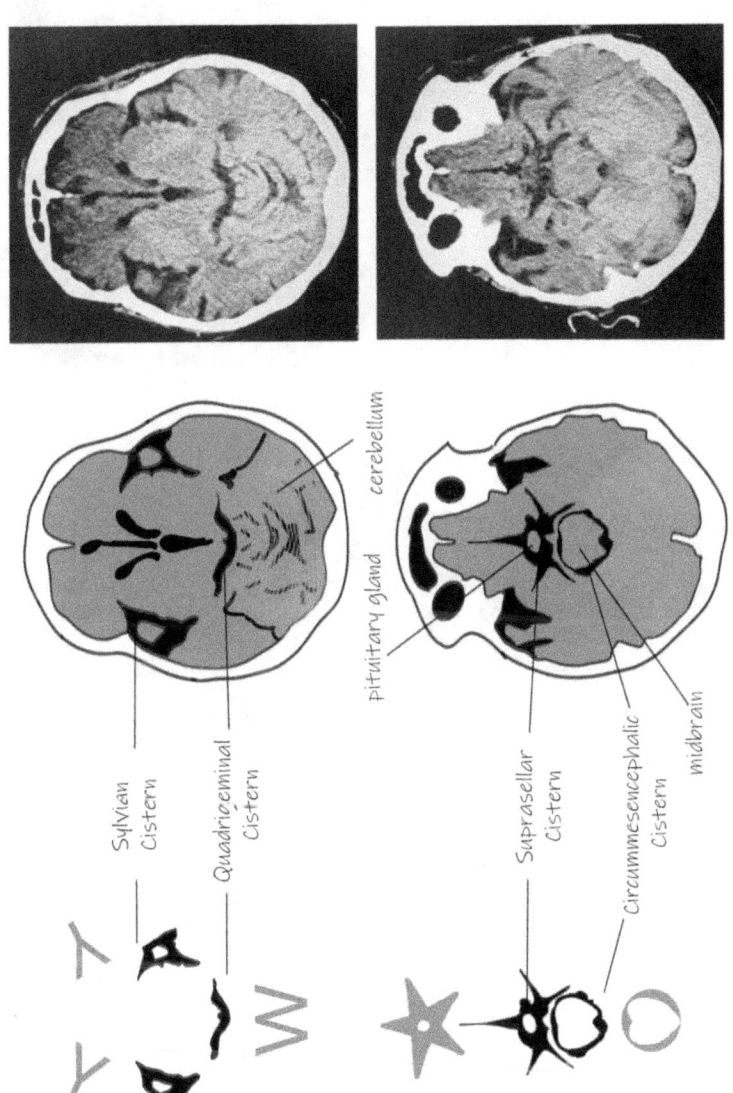

cerebellum

Sylvian Cistern

Quadrigeminal Cistern

pituitary gland

Suprasellar Cistern

Circummesencephalic Cistern

midbrain

The white starfish sign indicates hemorrhage in the suprasellar cistern. this is an ominous sign of brain aneurysm rupture that appears in about 80% of subarachnoid hemorrhages cases. Don't forget that the suprasellar cistern is in proximity of the circle of Willis, which is the most common site of rupture of brain aneurysm. Notice in this picture the fresh clotted blood appears also in the sylvian cistern.

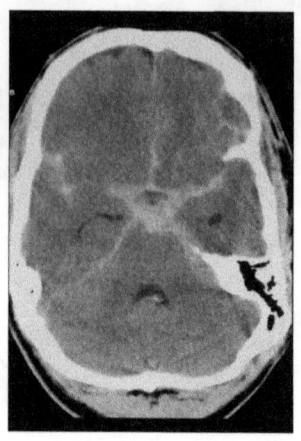

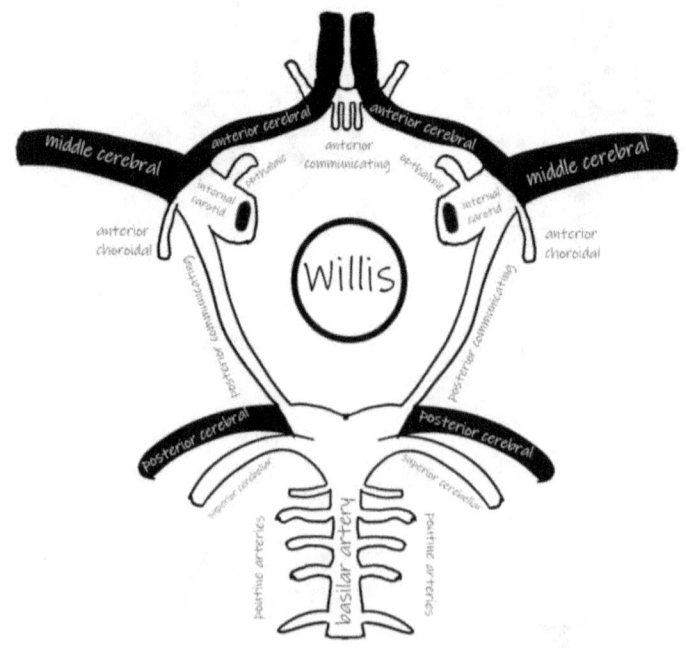

BRAIN

Normal finding: The brain matter normally appears as a hyperdense outer grey matter (light colored) and a hypodense inner white matter (dark color). The differentiation between these structures is vital in diagnosing ischemic stroke.

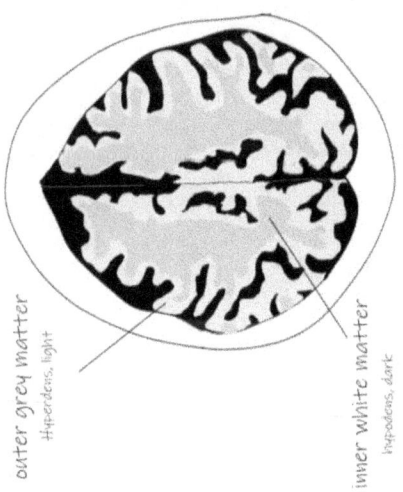

normal appearance of brain paranchyma
notice the good grey-white differentiation

outer grey matter
Hyperdens, light

inner white matter
hypodens, dark

Ischemic stroke (more common than hemorrhagic stroke)

Infarction appears darker than surrounding brain tissue. Other signs of parenchymal changes are

- loss of grey-white differentiation
- swelling or brain oedema appears as loss of curves of the grey matter on the brain surface (loss of the gyri).
- mass effect (compression of the ventricles and loss of symmetry) are seen within 12-14 hours.

Asymmetry and Midline shift of brain structures are important sign of pathology that should always draw your attention to the opposite side of the shift. Usually you would find a mass, haemorrhage or abscess, etc. Metastasis or tumors are usually well-defined round masses. Abscess may show air-fluid level.

ischemic stroke

loss of the gyri

darker ischemic area

loss of grey-white differentiation

the occipital lobe of the lateral ventricle disappeared

compression of the frontal horn of the lateral ventricle

slight midline shift

Middle Cerebral Artery (MCA) Hyperdense sign

Early sign of ischemic stroke is seen within 2-4 hours is the Middle Cerebral Artery (MCA) Hyperdense sign, where a fresh blood clot may be formed. Look for this sign at the level of the suprasellar cistern.

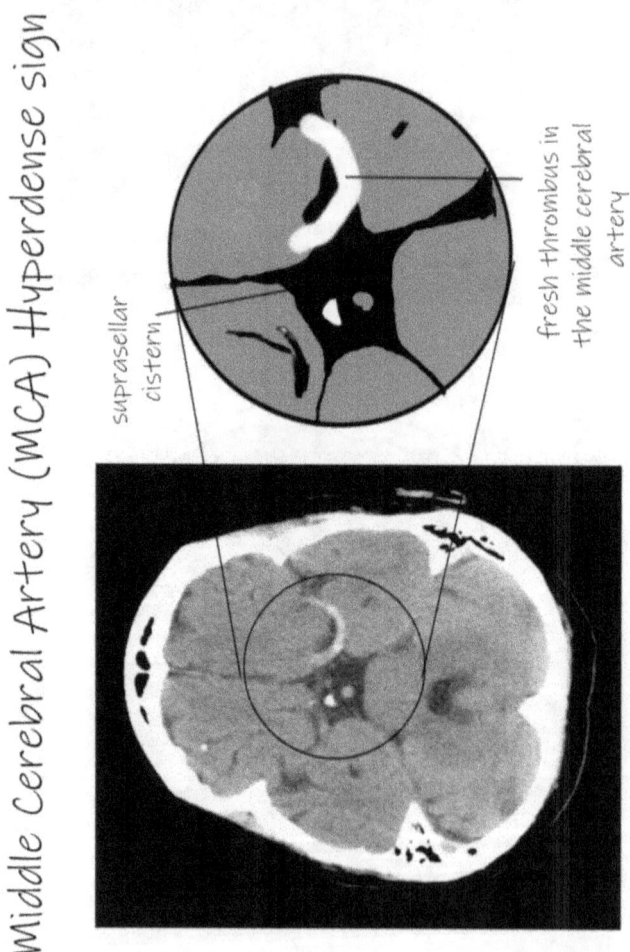

Middle Cerebral Artery (MCA) Hyperdense sign

suprasellar cistern

fresh thrombus in the middle cerebral artery

Ventricles

Normal findings: Ventricles appears as fluid (CSF) filled hypodense structures within the brain parenchyma. Hyperdense bodies may appear inside the ventricles. These are normal calcifications in lateral ventricles (pineal body and choroid plexus).

Lateral ventricles	2 back to back commas
Third ventricle	Slit-shaped
Fourth ventricle	Helmet-shaped

- Look for blood inside the ventricles which may appear as a blood-fluid level.
- Collapse of a ventricle or a midline shit is due to a space-occupying lesion in the adjacent parenchyma (bleeding or tumor).
- Slit-shaped ventricles bilaterally with loss of the gyri is a sign of diffuse axonal injury (brain oedema) due to rapid deceleration injury (car accident)

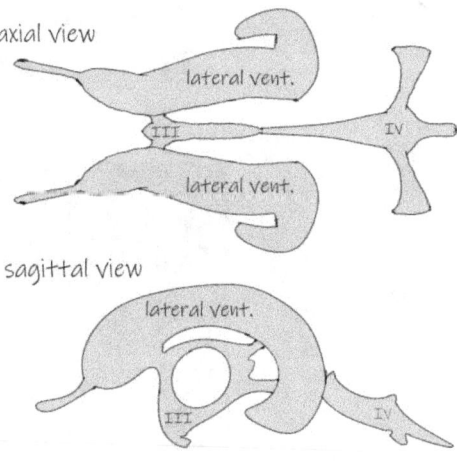

axial view

lateral vent.

III   IV

lateral vent.

sagittal view

lateral vent.

III   IV

Brain Ventricles

lateral ventricles

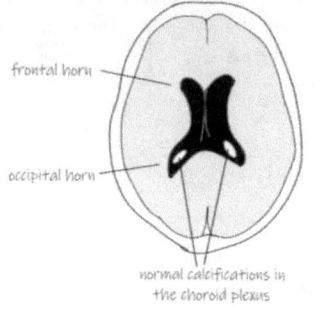

frontal horn

occipital horn

normal calcifications in
the choroid plexus

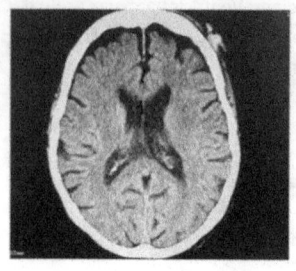

lateral ventricle

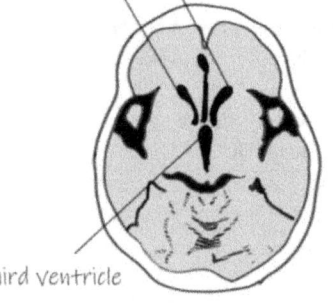

third ventricle

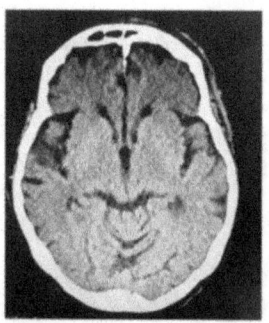

fourth ventricle

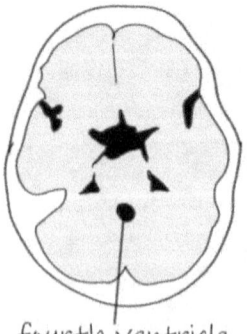

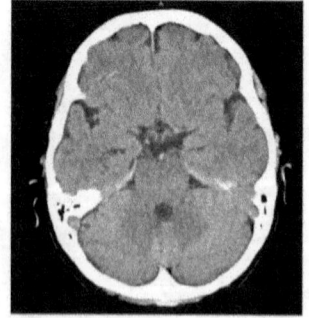

BONE (BONE WINDOW)

Look for soft tissue swelling, blood in sinuses or mastoid air cells, widened of skulls sutures or visible fractures. Notice in the picture below that skull fracture is only visible in the bone window.

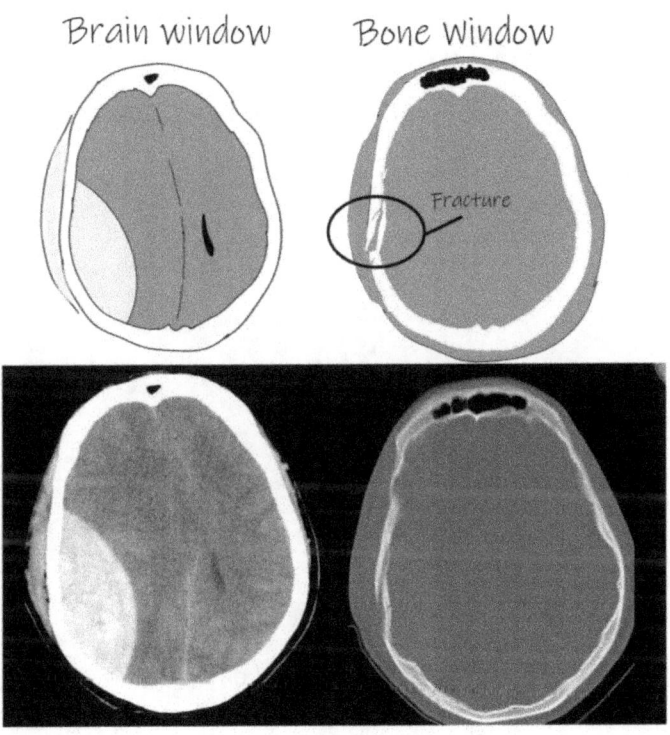

CONCLUSION

IF

- ✓ you did not see blood anywhere

- ✓ All cisterns are present and opened

- ✓ The brain is symmetric with normal grey-white matter differentiation

- ✓ The ventricles are symmetrical without dilation

- ✓ No fractures seen

THEN

There is no emergent diagnosis from the CT scan.

CHAPTER 6

SKELETAL X-RAYS

Contents

General concepts in evaluating skeletal X-Rays	74
Pelvis	76
Knee joint	80
Ankle joint	84
Foot	88
Shoulder joint	92
Elbow joint	96
Wrist joint and Hand	100
Lumbar vertebrae	104
Cervical vertebrae	108

GENERAL CONCEPTS IN EVALUATING SKELETAL X-RAYS

To evaluate any skeletal x-ray, you must check at first its quality. There are three main questions that you should always ask before beginning your evaluation.

I.   Is the data accurate?

Is this the right patient? The right date? And the right side to be investigated?

II.   Does everything visible?

There are standard requirements of every x-ray in which a minimum of structures should be visible to evaluate it thoroughly. For example, a long bone x-ray should always include at least one joint in the view. Another example, the hand x-ray. All fingers and the wrist joint should be clearly visible. Don't accept an x-ray with technical failures like an earing blocking the view of a part of cervical vertebrae or a missing little toe in a foot x-ray.

III.   Does everything correctly align?

Malrotation can dramatically hinder the ability to spot a fracture or a dislocation. Also, malrotation affect all measurement of distances and angles of x-rays rendering these valuable tools useless.

Features of bony fractures seen in plain x-ray.

I.   Primary features

a.   Gapping and dislocation: presence of a gap in a bony shaft with or without dislocation is the most obvious feature of a fracture.

b.   Cortical interruption: this is also a very reliable feature of a fracture. It advised to check every cortex of every visible bone on an x-ray film to exclude fractures. Non-dislocated or impacted fractures may present with only cortical interruption.

II.   Secondary features

a. Asymmetry: in comparison with the other side.

b. abnormal position: loss of alignment or shifting from the normal axis.

c. periosteal response: haziness of the area around the fracture due to periosteal effusion.

d. trabecular interruption: very prominent feature in fractures of the neck of the femur.

e. changes versus old images: especially useful in judging x-rays of older patients suffering from severe degenerative disorders or in patient with old fractures with a suspicious refracture.

In the next pages you will find the most common x-rays encountered in the emergency room setting. For each region you will see a diagram showing the basic radiological anatomy followed by the most common sites of fractures and a systematic way to judge this x-ray.

PELVIS

RADIOLOGICAL ANATOMY

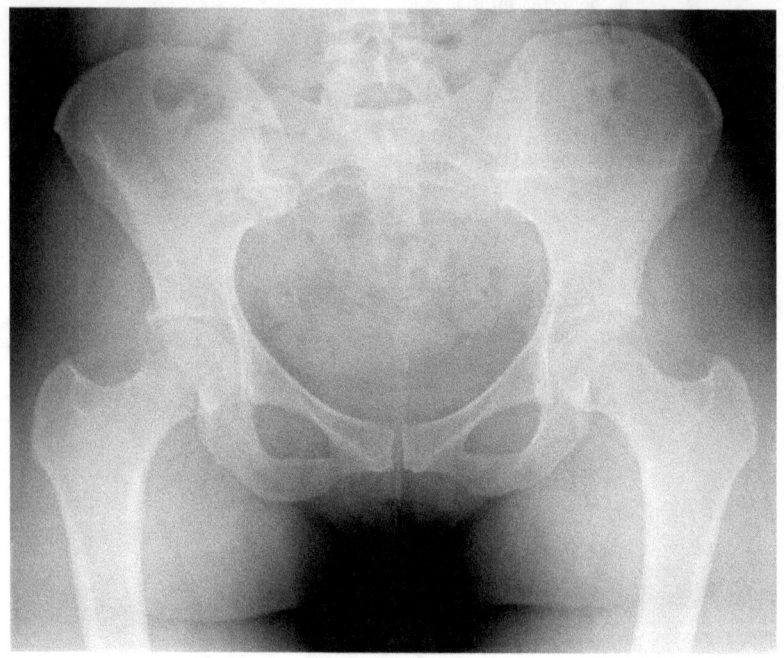

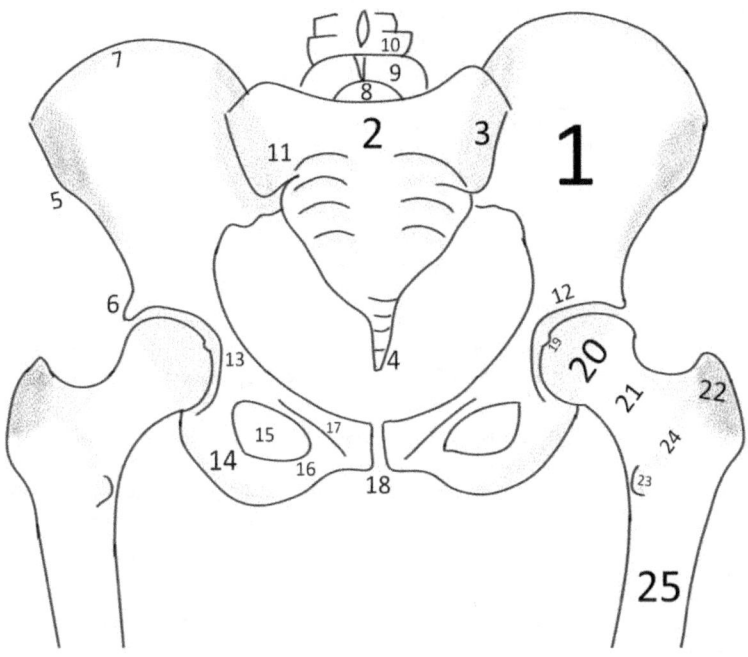

1.	Ileum	15.	Obturator foramen
2.	Sacrum	16.	Inferior pubic ramus
3.	Sacroiliac joint	17.	Superior pubic ramus
4.	Coccyx	18.	Symphysis pubis
5.	Anterior superior iliac spine	19.	Fovea
6.	Anterior inferior iliac spine	20.	Head of Femur
7.	Iliac crest	21.	Neck of femur
8.	Lumbo-sacral joint	22.	Greater trochanter
9.	5th lumbar vertebra	23.	Lesser trochanter
10.	4th lumbar vertebra	24.	Intertrochanteric ridge
11.	Sacral ala	25.	Femur shaft
12.	Acetabulum		
13.	Ischial spine		
14.	Ischial tuberosity		

Pelvic fracture	1	Trace the continuity of the pelvic ring and the obturator foramen for signs of pelvic fractures. Superior and inferior pubic rami are common sites of anterior pelvic fractures.
	2	Confirm the normal appearance of the sacroiliac joint which is a common site of posterior pelvic fractures.
	3	Check the acetabulum for fractures.
Fracture of the neck of the femur	4	Check the neck of femur, greater and lesser trochanter for proximal femur fractures. Look for cortical as well as trabecular interruption.
	5	Shenton's line: any deformity of this line may indicate a fractur of the neck of the femur. This is a imaginary line passing through the inferior border of the superior pubic ramus and the medial side of the neck of femur. normal contour of this line doesn't exclude a fracture.
Avulsion fractures	6	Check the anterior superior/inferior iliac spines for avulsion fractures.

Shenton's line:

In other words; don't trust a normal Shenton's line. It is only a good positive. Deformed Shenton's line without apparent fracture indicates a subtle fracture. That is it!

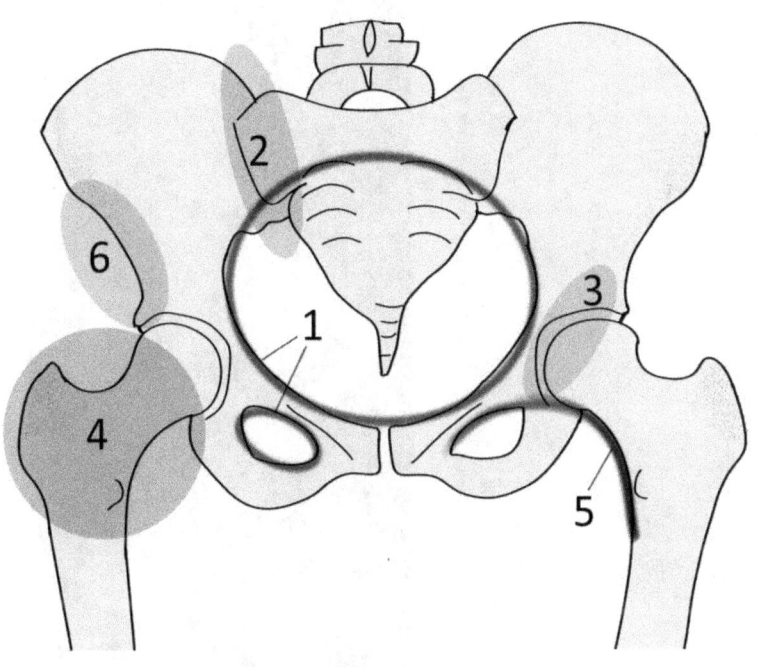

Knee joint

Radiological anatomy

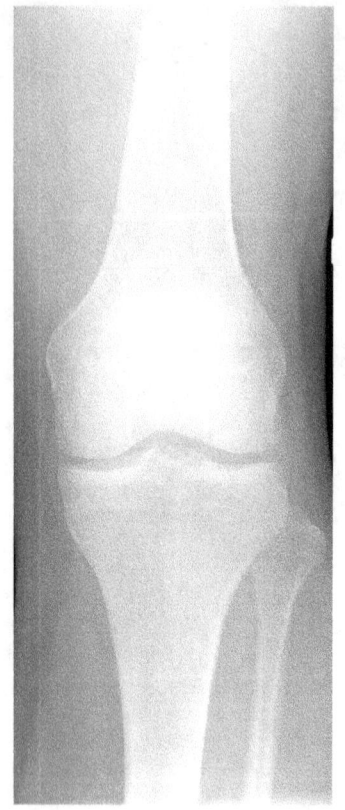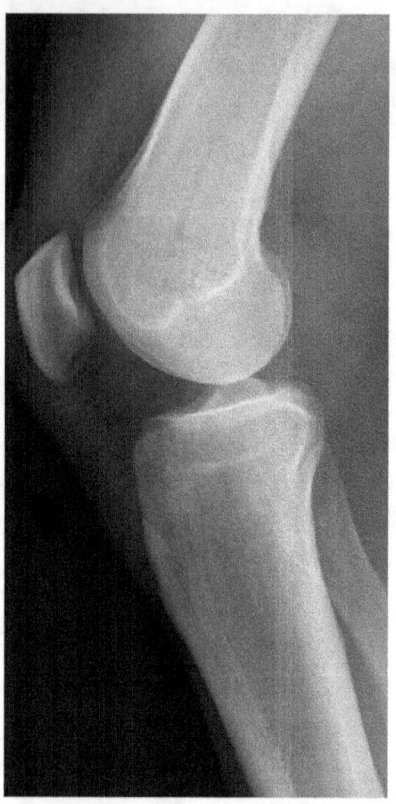

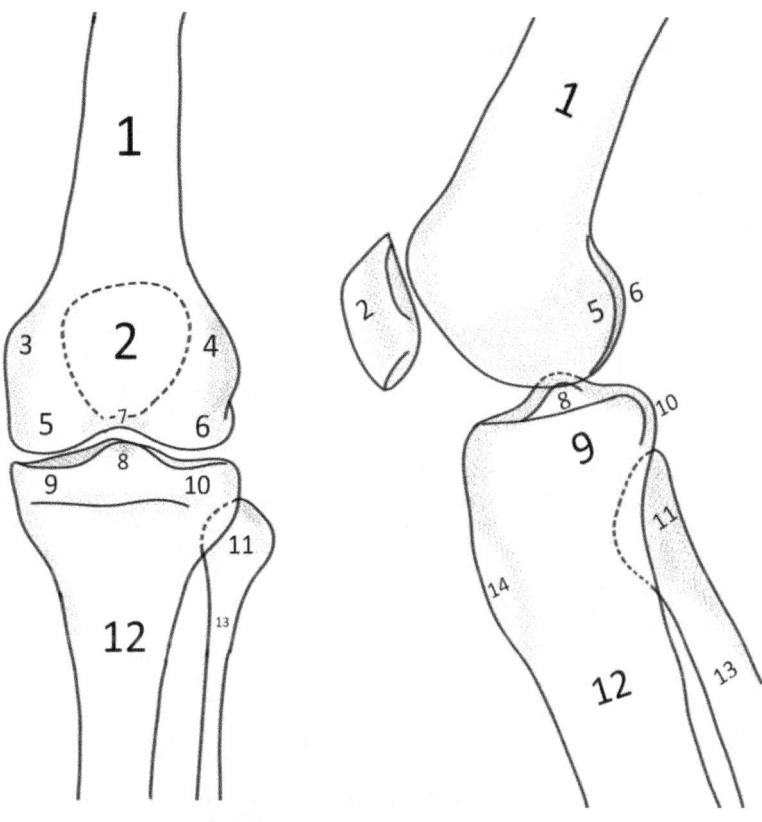

1.	Femur	8.	Intercondylar eminence
2.	Patella	9.	Medial tibial condyle
3.	Medial epicondyle	10.	Lateral tibial condyle
4.	Lateral epicondyle	11.	Head of fibula
5.	Medial femur condyle	12.	Tibia
6.	Lateral femur condyle	13.	Fibula
7.	Intercondylar notch	14.	Tibial tuberosity

Femur fracture	1	Check for supracondylar fracture.
Tibia fracture	2	Check for lateral and medial fracture.
Fibula fracture	3	Check for Maisonneuve fracture specially associated with ankle injury.
Patella dislocation	4	Confirm the normal position of patellar shadow to exclude patellar lateral dislocation.
Normal findings	5	A small sesamoid bone (Famella) may be present in this area.
Soft tissue injury	6	This a common site for seeing a hematoma. The clear distinction between blood and fatty tissue called the FBI sign (Fat-Blood Interface).
Cruciate ligament injury	7	The extension of an imaginary line extending between the roof the intercondylar notch of the femur (a) and the Intercondylar eminence (b) should be always to the posterior cortex of the tibia (c). inclination of this line indicate deviation of the longitudinal axis the knee joint due to a possible cruciate ligament injury. MRI is the diagnostic test.
Quadriceps or patellar tendon rupture.	8	A bony fragment in this area may indicate an avulsion fracture of the quadriceps tendon.
	9	The direction of patellar dislocation in patellar tendon rupture.
	10	The direction of patellar dislocation in quadriceps tendon rupture.
	11	Blumensaat line is the line drawn along the roof of the intercondylar notch of the femur as seen on lateral radiograph of the knee joint. It can been used for indicating the relative position of the patella as normally this line intersects the lower pole of the patella.
	12	To asses patellar deviation compare the area of contact between the patella and femur (d) and the perpendicular distance between the lower pole of the patella (e) and the flat surface of the tibia. A ratio more the one indicates patellar dislocation.

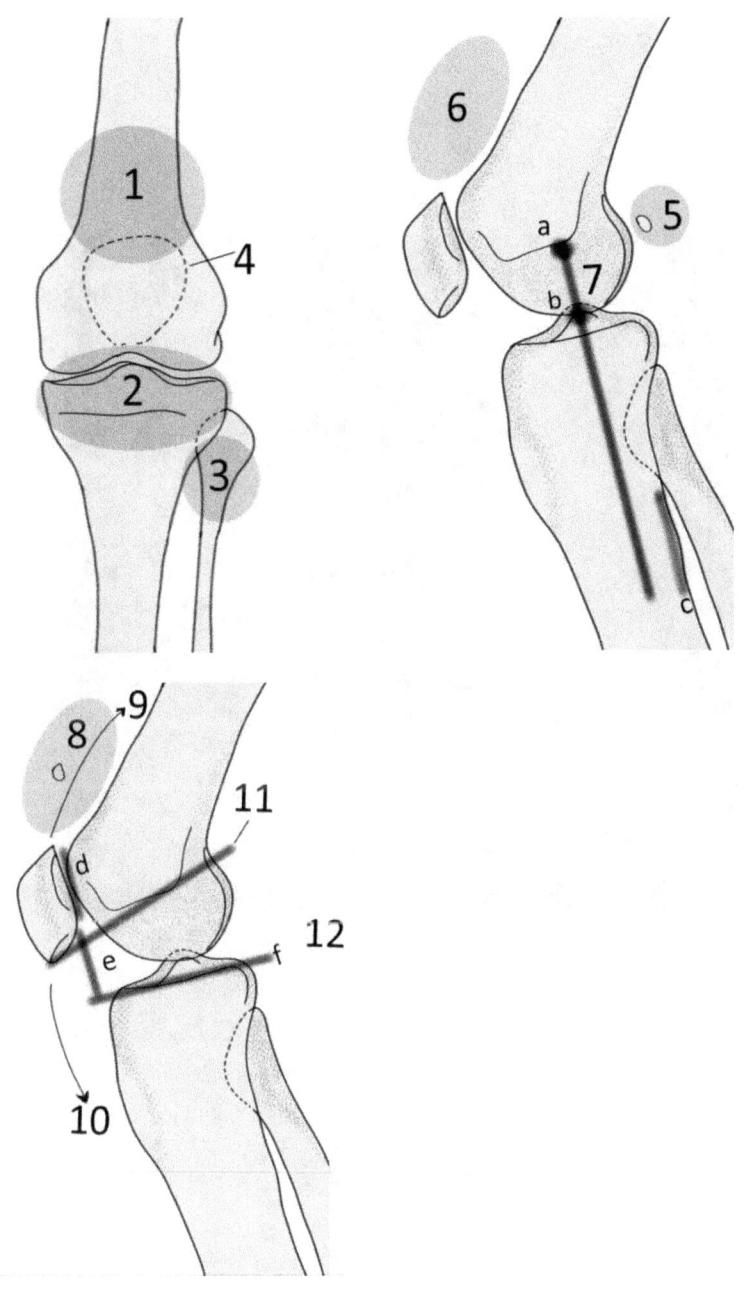

ANKLE JOINT

RADIOLOGICAL ANATOMY

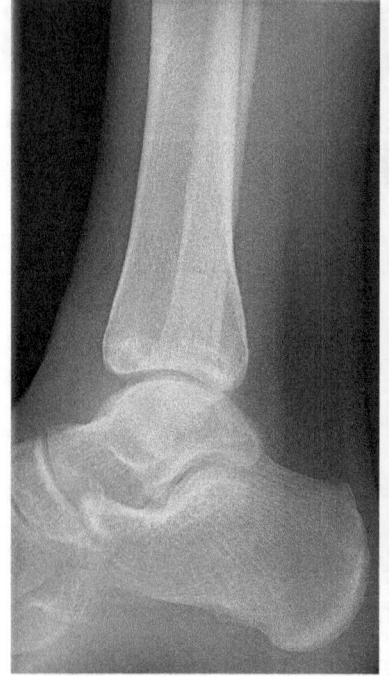 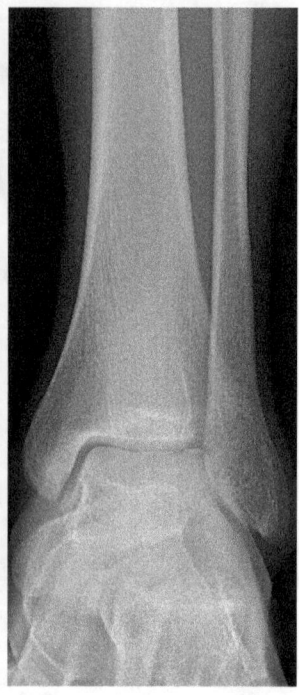

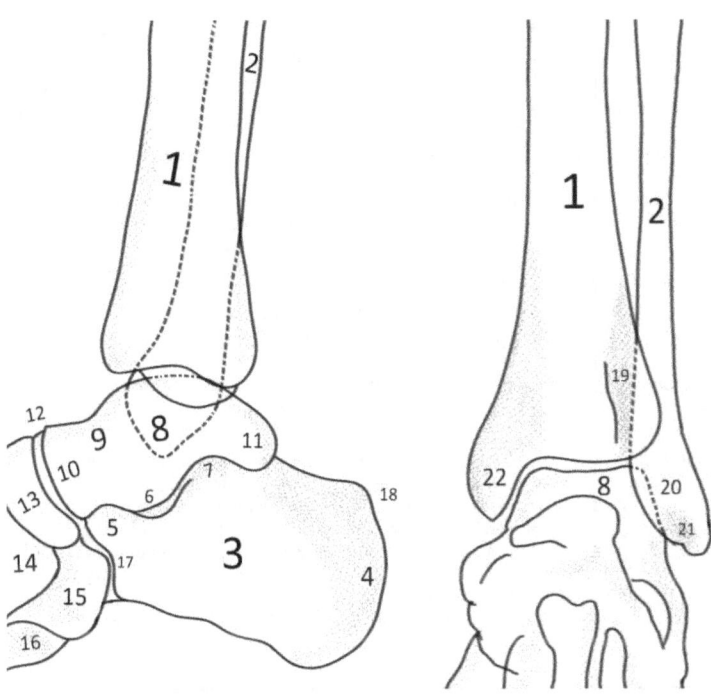

1.	Tibia	12.	Talonavicular joint
2.	Fibula	13.	Navicular
3.	Calcaneus	14.	Medial cuneiform
4.	Calcaneal tuberosity	15.	Cuboid
5.	Anterior process	16.	Base of the 5th metatarsal
6.	Sinus tarsi	17.	Calcaneocuboid joint
7.	Talocalcaneal joint	18.	Achilles tendon insertion
8.	Talus body	19.	Fibular notch
9.	Talus neck	20.	Lateral malleolus
10.	Talus head	21.	Malleolar fossa
11.	Posterior process	22.	Medial malleolus

Lateral malleolus fracture	1	Check for a fracture and its level in comparison with the syndesmoses.
Medial malleolus fracture	2	Check for a medial malleolar fracture sometimes associated with a lateral malleolar fracture. Also look in this area for avulsion fracture associated with deltoid ligament injury.
Syndesmotic injury	3	Check the width of the tibiofibular overlap area (a). This should be measured 1 cm above the tibial plafond. Normally it should be more than 6 mm in anteroposterior images. A smaller area of overlap indicates a widened tibiofibular space, which by turn is an indicator of a syndesmotic injury.
	4	A uniform tibiotalar joint space that measures 3 to 4 mm indicates an intact syndesmosis.
Posterior malleolus fracture	5	Check a fracture at the Volkmann's triangle specially in association of a bimalleolar fracture.
Calcaneal fracture	6	Bohler's angle: is the angle between the anterior and the posterior plane of the calcaneus. The anterior plane is represented by a line between the top of the anterior process (d) and the dome of the calcaneus (c), while the posterior plane is represented by a line drawn between the superior end of the calcaneal tuberosity (b) and the dome of the calcaneus (c). This angle is normally between 20° and 40°. A deviation from these values is an evidence of calcaneal fracture.

Normal values:
width of the tibiofibular
overlap: > 6 mm
tibiotalar joint space: 3-4
mm
Bohler's angle: 20°-40°

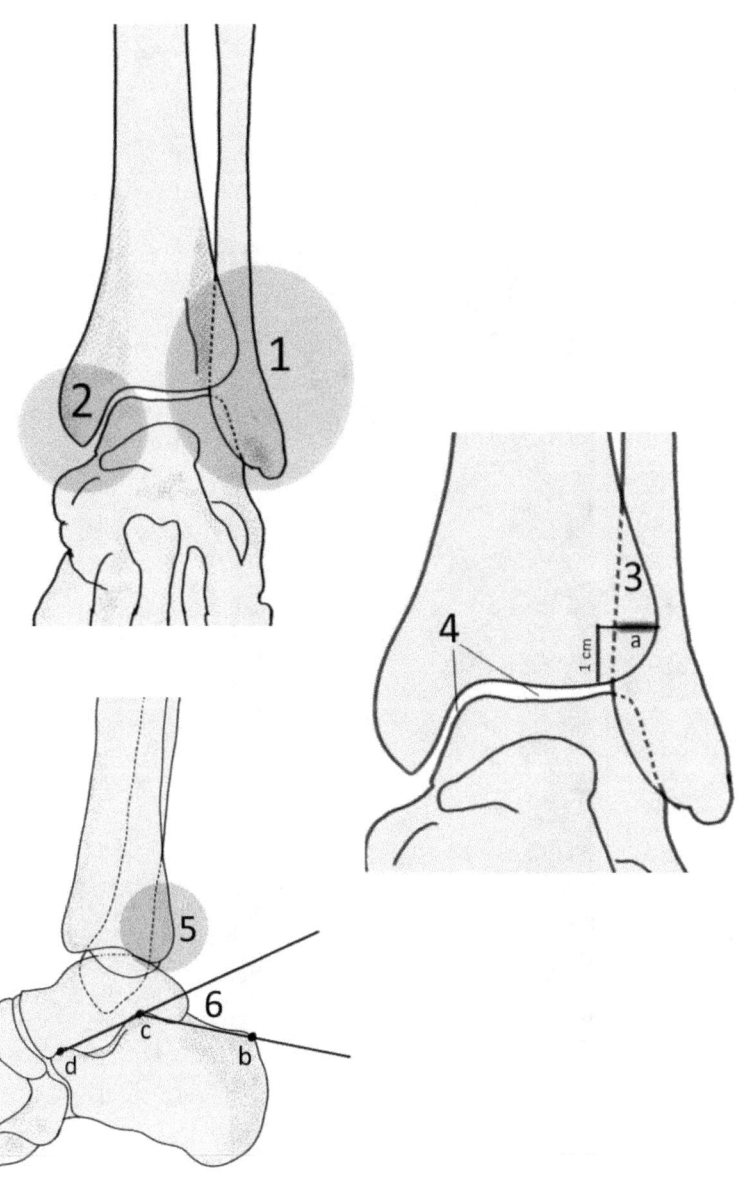

FOOT

RADIOLOGICAL ANATOMY

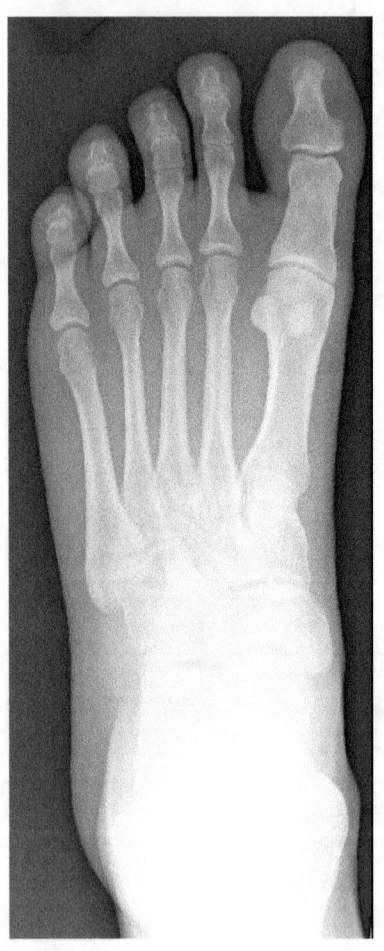

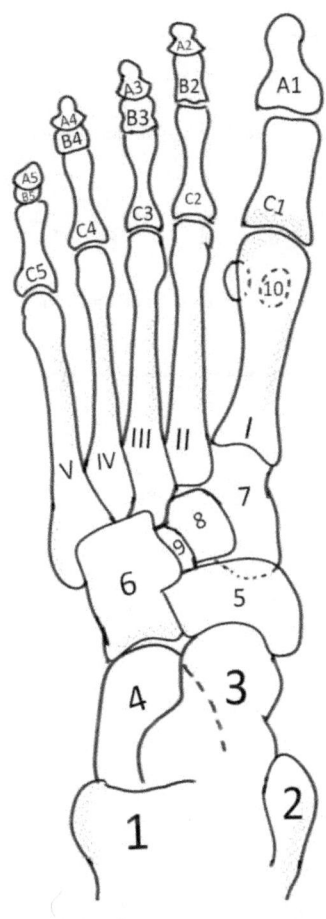

1. Tibia	10. Sesamoid bone
2. Fibula	A1-A5. Distal phalanges
3. Talus	B2-B5. Intermediate phalanges
4. Calcaneum	C1-C5. Proximal phalanges
5. Navicular	I-V. 1st to 5th metatarsals
6. Cuboid	
7. Medial cuneiform	
8. Intermediate cuneiform	
9. Lateral cuneiform	

Proximal 5th metatarsal fracture	1	The most common foot fracture, associated with ankle joint sprain.
5th Toe proximal phalanx and distal 5th metatarsal fracture	2	A common site for dislocation fracture.
Big toe	3	Both phalanges are site of fracture caused by direct trauma.
Proximal 2nd to 4th metatarsal fractures	4	Caused by exaggerated plantarflexion.

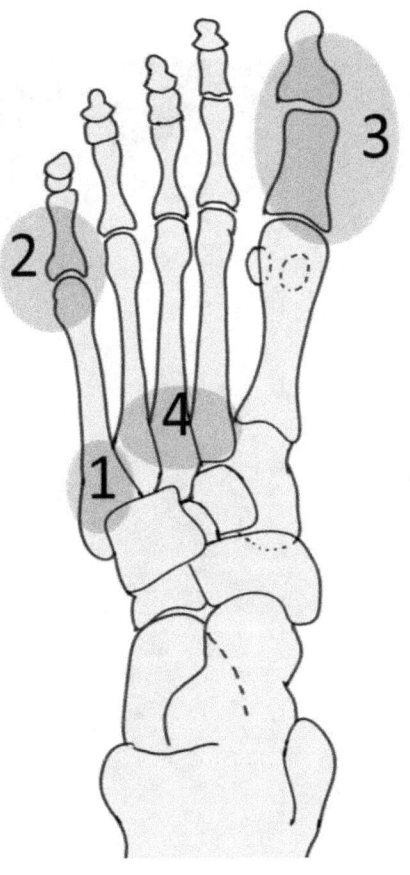

SHOULDER JOINT

RADIOLOGICAL ANATOMY

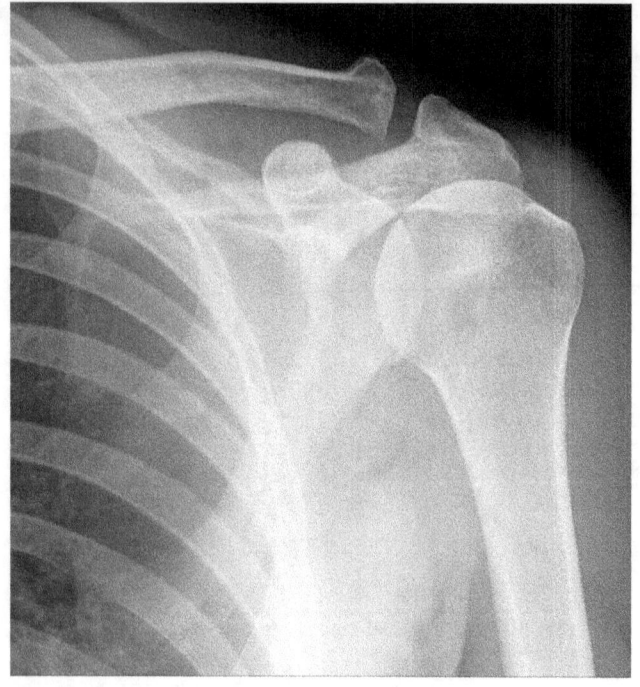

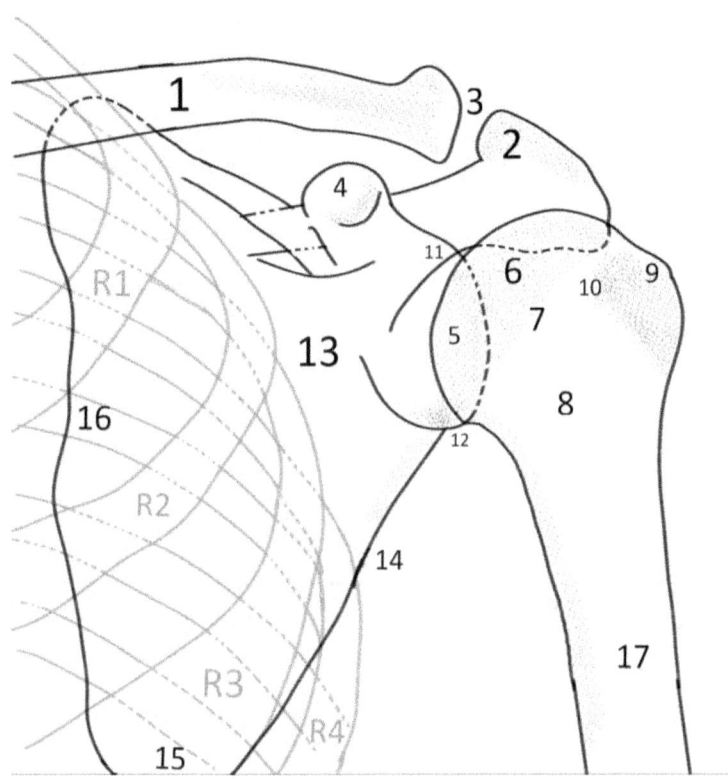

1.	Clavicle	10.	Lesser tuberosity
2.	Acromion process	11.	Supraglenoid tubercle
3.	Acromioclavicular joint	12.	Infraglenoid tubercle
4.	Coracoid process	13.	Scapula
5.	Glenoid cavity	14.	Lateral border of scapula
6.	Head of the humerus	15.	Inferior angle
7.	Anatomical neck	16.	Medial border of scapula
8.	Surgical neck	17.	Shaft of the humerus
9.	Greater tuberosity	R1 – R4. Anterior rips 1 to 4	

Clavicular fracture	1	Look here for a clavicular fracture. This is a common fracture. The proximal fragment is normally superiorly dislocated by the pulling action of the sternomastoid muscle, while the distal fragment is inferiorly dislocated as it is pulled down by the weight of the arm.
Acromioclavicular joint dislocation	2	Asses the level of the clavicle in relation to the acromion. An elevated clavicular lateral end indicates an Acromioclavicular joint dislocation.
Humerus neck fracture	3	Check the proximal humerus for a fracture at the anatomical neck (b) or more common at the surgical neck (a).
Shoulder dislocation	4	Abnormal position of the head of the humerus indicates a dislocation. More than 90% of dislocation are anterior dislocation. It is important to check for an accompanying fracture before trying a reposition. The distance between a head of the humerus and the acromion (c) is normally between 7 and 11 mm. a wider distance indicates a dislocation.
Greater tuberosity avulsion fracture	5	Check this area for an avulsion of the greater tuberosity,

Normal values:
Acromio-humeral distance: 7-11 mm.

✓ Greater distance (> 11 mm) indicates a shoulder dislocation.

✓ Smaller distance (< 7 mm) indicates a rotator cuff injury (mostly chronic injury).

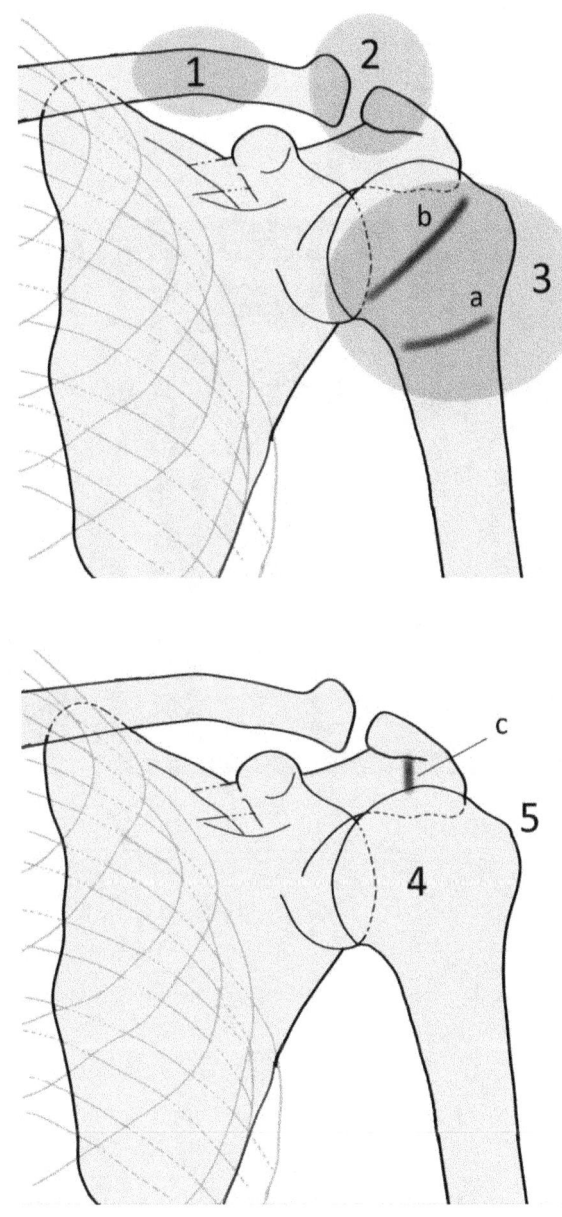

ELBOW JOINT

RADIOLOGICAL ANATOMY

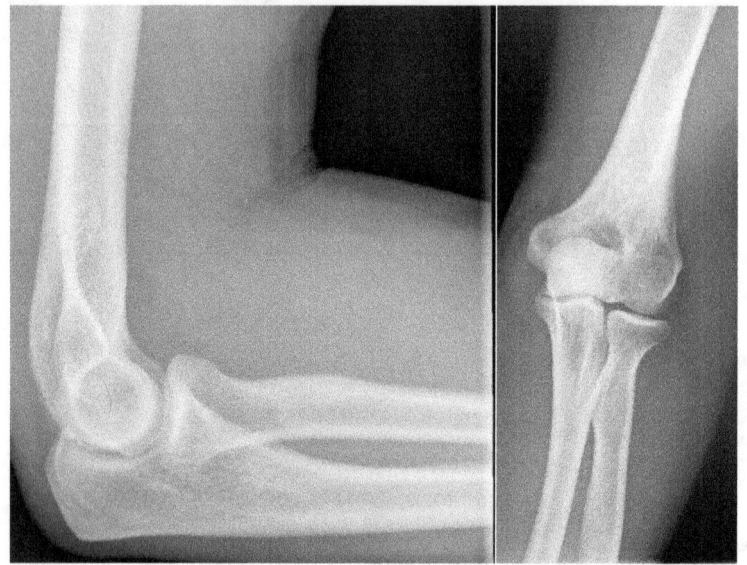

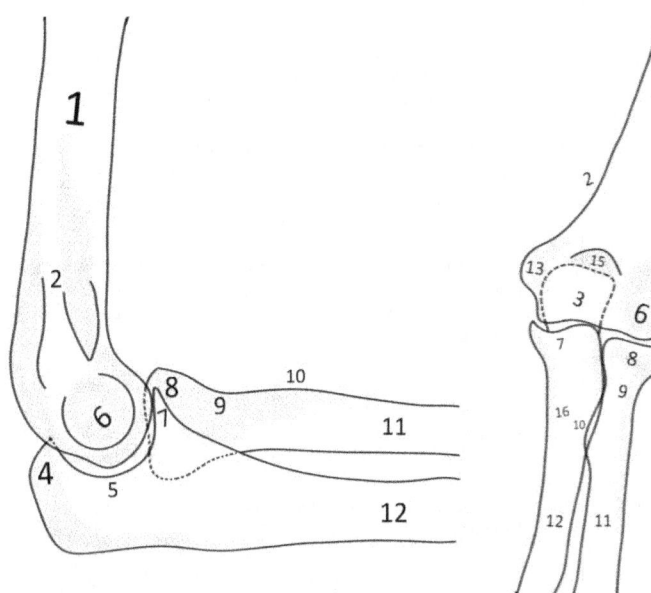

1. Humerus shaft
2. Supracondylar ridge
3. Trochlea
4. Olecranon process
5. Trochlear notch
6. Capitulum
7. Coronoid process
8. Head of radius
9. Neck of radius
10. Radial tuberosity
11. Radius shaft
12. Ulnar shaft
13. Medial epicondyle
14. Lateral epicondyle
15. Olecranon fossa
16. Ulnar tuberosity

Alignment	1	Correct alignment is crucial to judge other aspects of elbow x-ray. This is determined by the presence of a clear figure of "8" formed by the cortical marking of the supracondylar ridge and the capitulum.
Indirect sings of fractures	2	Visible pad of fat could indicate joint effusion caused by a fracture. The pad of fat appears as a darker area (radiolucent) surrounded by normally lighter (radiopaque) soft tissue. Anterior pad of fat (a) could be normally found as a thin shadow. Pathological enlarged anterior pad of fat is called: Sail sign. Posterior pad of fat is always pathological.
	3	Anterior humerus line: passes along the anterior border of the distal humerus. It should always intersect the central part of the capitulum (c). Otherwise is an indication of a dislocation or a fracture.
	4	Radio-capitellar line: passes through the central part of proximal radial shaft. It should always intersect the capitulum and the anterior humerus line at the center of the capitulum (c). Otherwise is an indication of a dislocation or a fracture.
Proximal ulnar fracture	5	The olecranon process is the most common site of ulnar fracture.
Proximal radial fracture	6	Don't miss a fracture at the radius head. It could either clearly visible specially at the articular surface, or barely visible as a kink or slight abnormal angulation at or just above the neck of the radius (d).
Distal humeral fracture	7	A supracondylar humeral fracture is relatively common in children.

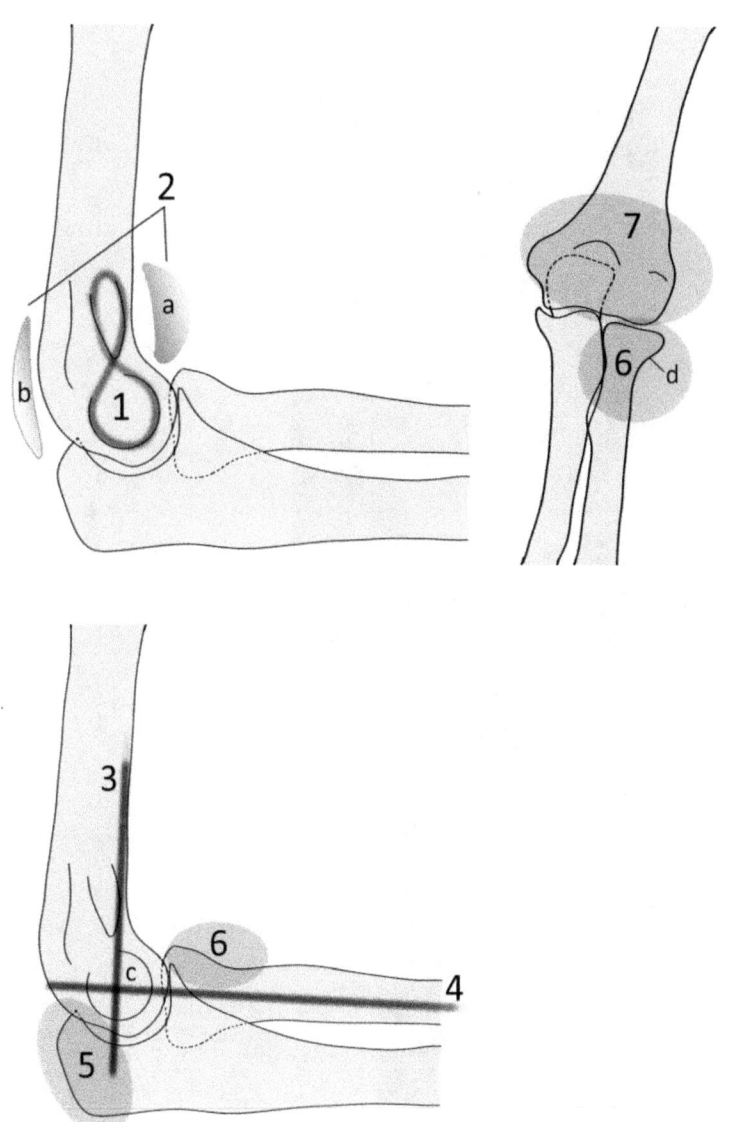

WRIST JOINT AND HAND

RADIOLOGICAL ANATOMY

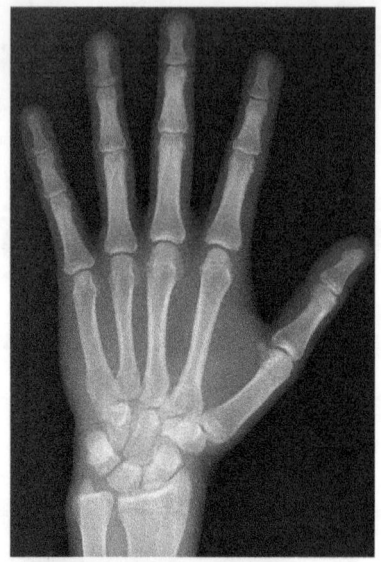

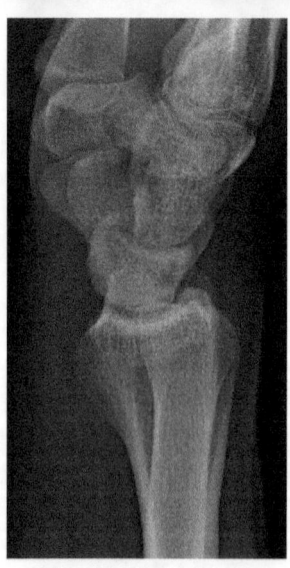

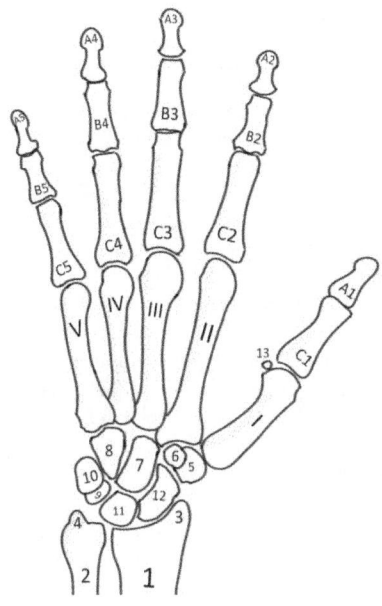

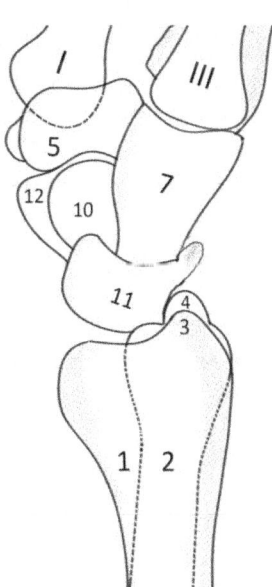

1.	Radius
2.	Ulna
3.	Styloid process (radius)
4.	Styloid process (ulna)
5.	Trapezium
6.	Trapezoid
7.	Capitate
8.	Hamate
9.	Triquetrum
10.	Pisiform
11.	Lunate
12.	Scaphoid
13.	Sesamoid bone

A1-A5. Distal phalanges
B2-B5. Intermediate phalanges
C1-C5. Proximal phalanges
I-V. 1st to 5th metacarpals

Metacarpal fractures	1	Boxer's fracture of the head of the 5th metacarpal.
	2	Fracture of the base of the 5th metacarpal.
	3	Rolando's fracture of the base of the 1st metacarpal.
Carpal fracture	4	Scaphoid fracture.
	5	Check the alignment of the capitate, lunate and the radius bone. Malalignment indicates either a perilunate dislocation (only the capitate is dislocated) or a lunate dislocation (only the lunate is dislocated).
	6	a bony fragment in this area indicates a possible triquetral avulsion fracture.
Radial and ulnar fractures	7	Check the contour of the radius for possible fractures
	8	Radial inclination: is the angle between a horizontal plane (a) perpendicular on the radial longitudinal axis (x) and a line drawn between the styloid process and the ulnar corner of the radius (b). normal value is 23°. Smaller angles are called radial tilt that indicates a fracture.
	9	Ulnar variance: is the longitudinal distance between a line tangential to the ulnar articular surface (c) and radius articular surface at the lunate fossa (a). Normal values are between 0 and 2 mm.
	10	Volar and dorsal tilt: is the angle between a horizontal plane (a) perpendicular on the radial longitudinal axis (x) and a line drawn between the styloid process and the ulnar corner of the radius (b). normal value is 11° volar tilt. Further inclination in the direction (d) is a pathological volar tilt. Inclination in the direction (e) is a dorsal tilt which is always pathological.

Normal values:
Radial inclination: 23°
Ulnar variance: 0-2 mm
Volar tilt: 11°
Dorsal tilt: -

AAOS guidelines of operative management*
✓ Radial shortening > 3mm
✓ Ulnar variance > 2mm
✓ Dorsal tilt > 10°
✓ Intra-articular displacement

* American Association of Orthopedic Surgeons

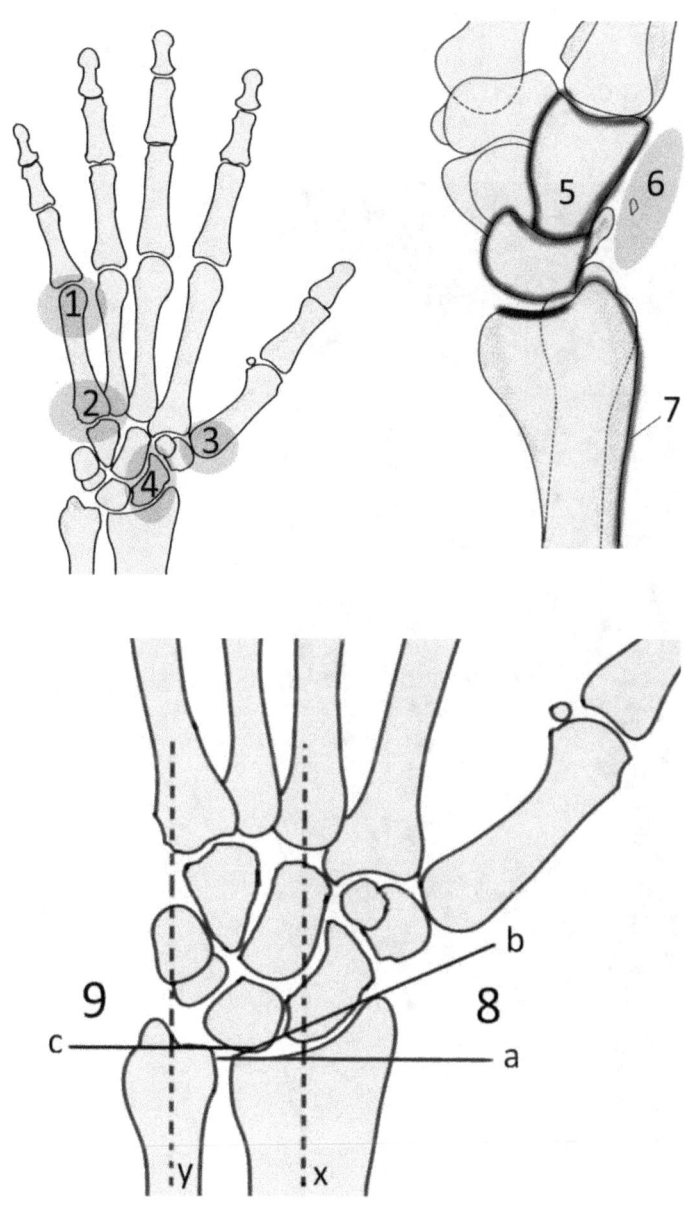

Lumbar vertebrae

Radiological anatomy

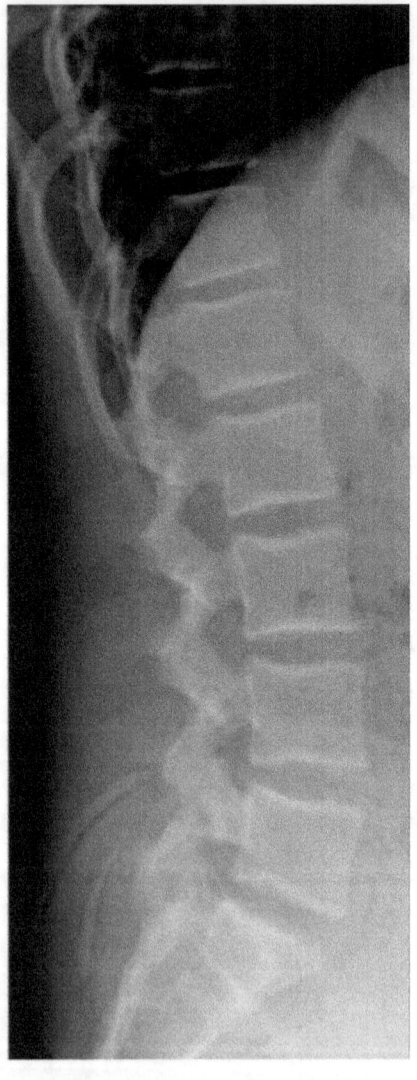

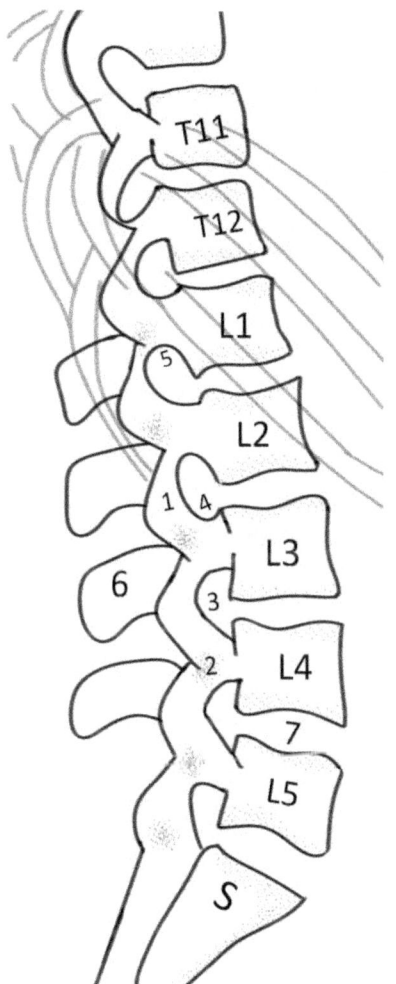

1.	Inferior articular process
2.	Pedicle
3.	Intervertebral foramen
4.	Inferior vertebral notch
5.	Superior vertebral notch
6.	Spinous process
7.	Intervertebral desc space
T11-12. thoracic vertebra	
L1 – L5. lumbar vertebrae	
S. Sacrum	

Leveling	1	Identify the 12th thoracic vertebra by the attachment of the last rip.
		Identify the last lumbar vertebra (5th or 6th) which is just above the sacrum.
		In 25% of the population a Lumbosacral transitional vertebra could be identified. It is an extra vertebra that could be considered to belong to sacral (sacralized L5 segment) or lumbar vertebrae (lumbarised S1 segment).
Alignment	2	Check the alignment of all visible vertebrae for dislocated or protruding vertebrae. Loss of alignment could be an indication of a fracture.
Vertebral height	3	Loss of height is an indication of a fracture.

3 common types of vertebral fractures

✓ Compression fracture: only loss of height without loss of alignment.

✓ Burst fracture: loss of both height and alignment (due to anterior protrusion of the fractured vertebra)

✓ Chance fracture: a horizontal fracture of the 3 columns of the vertebra with possible gaping of the spinal processes posteriorly.

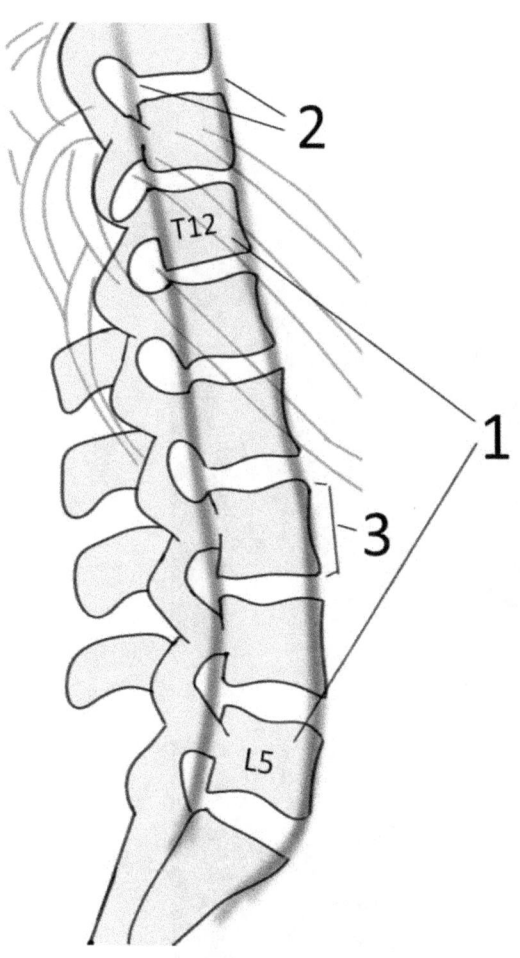

T12

L5

2

1

3

Cervical vertebrae

Radiological anatomy

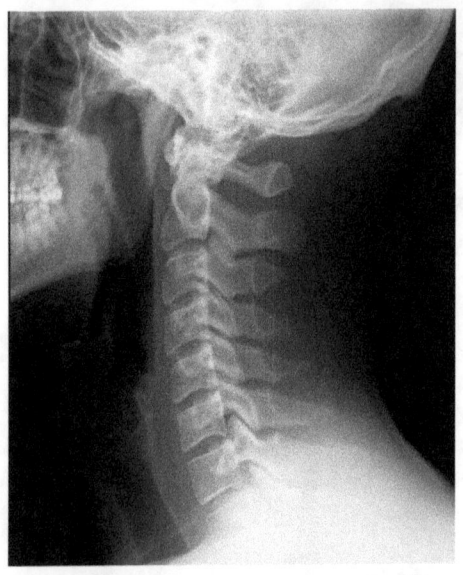

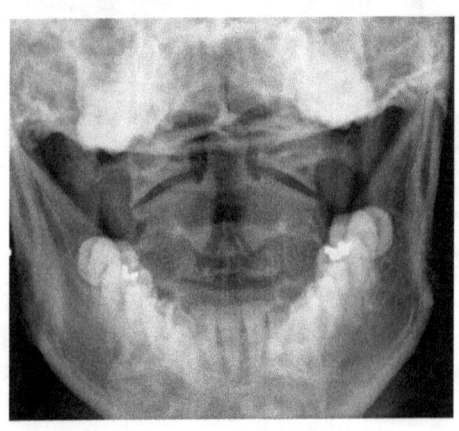

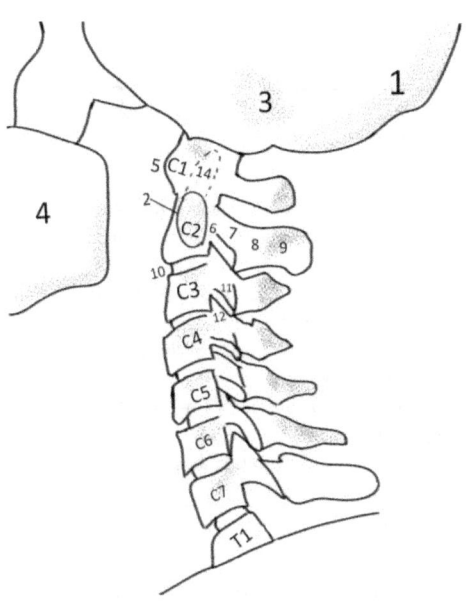

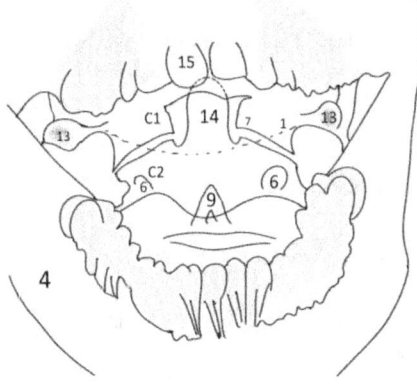

1.	Occiput
2.	Harris ring
3.	Mastoid air cells
4.	Mandible
5.	Anterior arch of C1
6.	Pedicle
7.	Lateral mass
8.	Lamina
9.	Spinous process
10.	Intervertebral desc space
11.	Superior facet
12.	Inferior facet
13.	Transverse process C1
14.	Odontoid process
15.	Central incisors

C1 – C7. Cervical vertebrae
T1. 1st thoracic vertebra

Leveling	1	Determine the level of C1 and T1. Both should be visible in an adequate cervical x-ray.
Alignment	2	Check the alignment of the cervical vertebrae for signs of dislocation or fractures through observing 3 longitudinal lines: (a) The anterior line formed by the anterior longitudinal ligament. (b) The posterior line formed by the posterior longitudinal ligament. (c) The spinolaminar line formed by the anterior edges of the spinous processes. Note that the spinal cord (x) lies between the posterior line and the spinolaminar line.
Vertebral height	3	Loss of height is an indication of a fracture. Note that this rule doesn't apply to C1 which lack a vertebral body.
Odontoid process fracture	4	Disruption or a step seen in the cortical ring at the level of C2 is an indicator of odontoid process fracture. This ring is formed the lateral masses of C2 viewed from the side. It is also known as Harris ring.
	5	Look for a visible fracture of the odontoid process.
	6	Lateral process should be aligned in the same plane.
	7	The spaces between the lateral masses of C1 and the odontoid process should be equal.

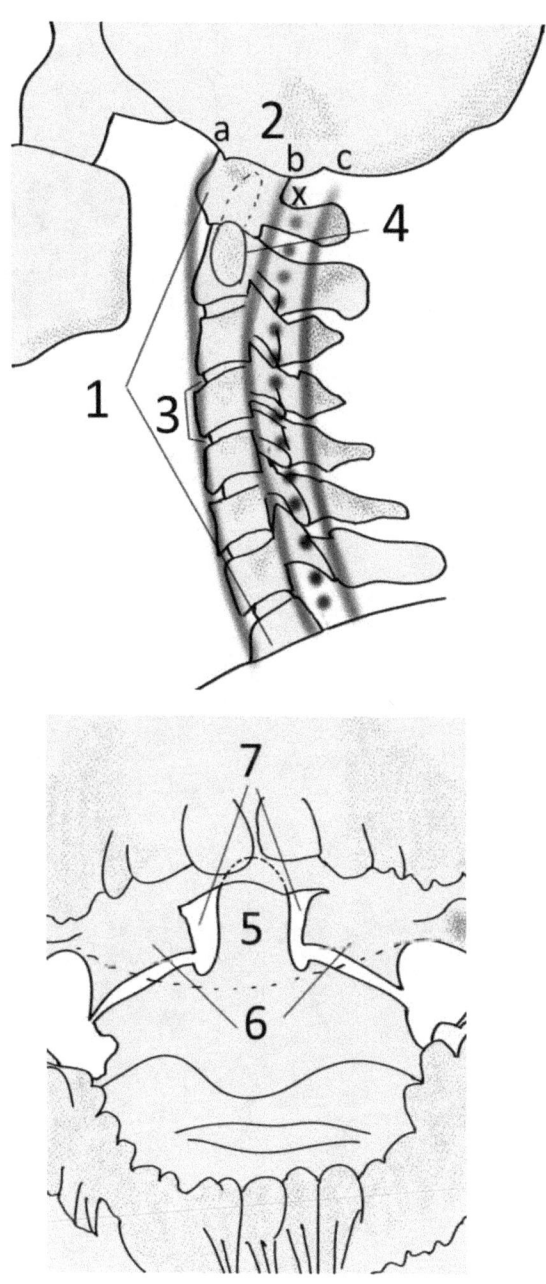

CHAPTER 7

EMERGENCY SONOGRAPHY (eFAST)

Contents

Introduction and basic concepts	113
Subxiphoid view	120
Inferior vena cava view	122
Right upper quadrant view	124
Left upper quadrant view	126
Pelvic sagittal view	128
Pelvic transversal view	130
Anterior thoracic view	132

INTRODUCTION AND BASIC CONCEPTS

FAST vs. eFAST

FAST is the famous acronym that stands for *Focused Assessment with Sonography for Trauma*. The aim of the FAST ultrasound scan is to rapidly detect the presence of blood in vital body cavities in the emergency room. This means rapidly detecting free fluid in pericardium, pleural space and peritoneum.

The more recent version of the FAST is the eFAST, which means extended FAST. In eFAST in addition to the previous aims, the detection of pneumothorax and hypovolemia is also included.

ANECHOIC, HYPERECHOIC AND HYPOECHOIC

As in most imaging techniques, the images obtained through sonography are shades of grey. The intensity of the white color or the brightness of any structure depends on its ability to reflect the ultrasonic waves back to the probe. This ability varies also according to the nature of the structure itself.

According to this principle, structures can be seen bright or dark. Bright structures reflect more ultrasonic waves back (reflect more echo), so called hyperechoic. While darker structures reflect less echo, and called hypoechoic. Black structures don't reflect echo at all and are called anechoic. These are mostly fluid collections.

Mnemonic for tissues normal echogenicity

My Cat Loves Sunny Places

Most hypoechoic
(dark)

⬇

Most hyperechoic
(bright)

Medulla of the kidney
Cortex of the kidney
Liver
Spleen
Prostate

ORIENTATION: NEAR VS FAR FIELD

These are important terms to describe structures in the field of sonography. The near field represents the superficial structures (near to the probe), while the far field represents deep structures (far from the probe).

ORIENTATION: PROBE INDICATOR

In order to recognize structures relative positions in the field the probe must be correctly held. On every probe there is a marker (colored dot or an arrow according to the machine brand. This indicator always points to the right side of the image you see on the monitor. The standard position for abdominal scan is when the indicator is to the right in transverse scans and upwards in sagittal scans.

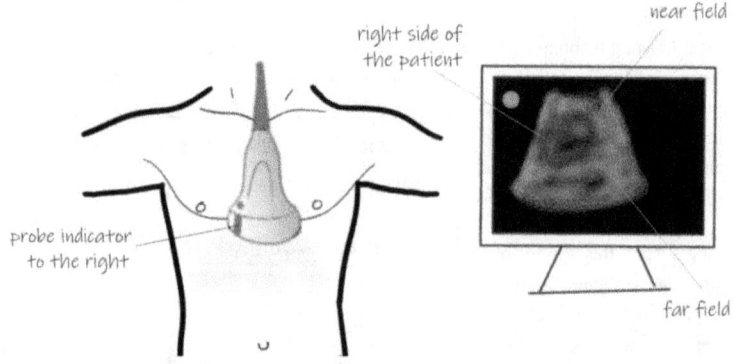

Free Fluid

The nature of any fluid could not be recognized using the ultrasound scan. But in the context of major trauma, any free fluid in body cavities is assumed to be blood.

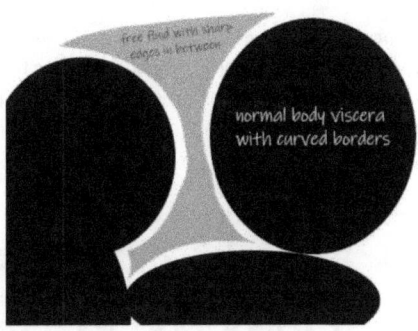

The abdomen is normally filled with different types of fluid. For example, gastric and intestinal content, blood running through blood vessels, bile waiting in the gall balder for a fatty meal or urine in the urinary bladder waiting for a decent WC. All this fluid appears in sonography anechoic (black). But they should not be mistaken for free fluid. The main difference is the shape of the fluid. Normal body fluids are always contained inside a viscus or a blood vessel. So, they always appear uniform shaped with curved borders. While free fluid in between these viscera accommodates the shape of the place between the curves and always shows sharp edges.

ACOUSTIC SHADOW

This phenomenon appears with solid structures. When ultrasonic waves hit a solid body (a bone or a stone in the gall bladder or the urinary tract) it can't penetrate it. So, it leaves a dark shadow beyond it, in which no echo returns to the probe. But the upper surface of this body appears bright or hyperechoic because almost all the waves are reflected on it.

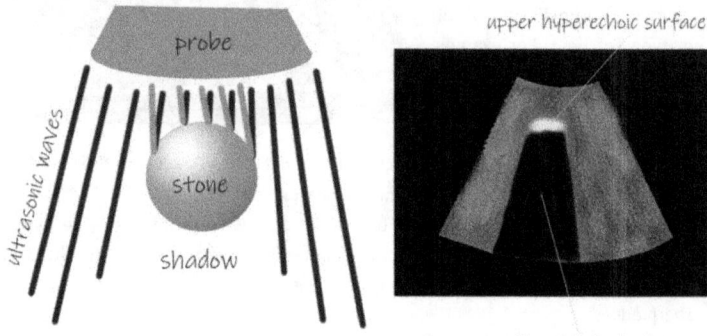

upper hyperechoic surface

acoustic anechoic shadow

MIRRORING ARTIFACT

The good inflated lung along with the diaphragm acts as mirror for the ultrasonic waves. Due to this mirroring effect, a reflected image of the liver and the spleen could be seen above the diaphragm. Loss of this effect indicates a fluid-filled lung field (due to pleural effusion for example).

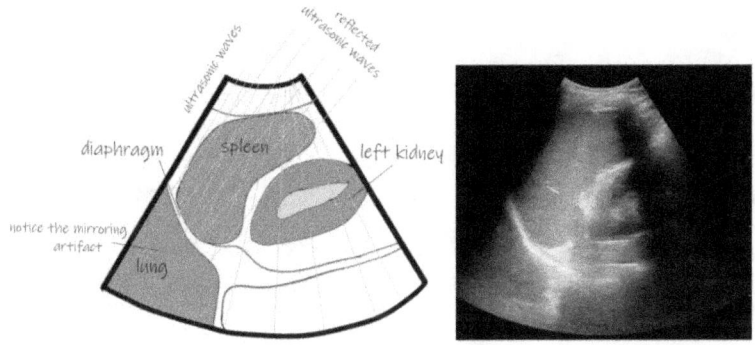

Basic views[5]

View	Site of the probe	Indicator towards Patient's	Visible structures	Expected pathology
Subxiphoid view (subcostal or pericardial)	Transverse under the xiphoid process	Right side	Liver Diaphragm Right and left sided chambers Lung	Absent or abnormal cardiac activity Pericardial fluid
Inferior Vena Cava view	Sagittal under the xiphoid process	Head	Liver Diaphragm Right atrium and ventricle IVC	Hypo- or Hypervolemia.
Right upper quadrant view (Perihepatic, Morison Pouch, or Right Flank View)	Coronal at right flank	Head	Liver Diaphragm Right kidney Hepatorenal space (Morison Pouch) Lung Spine	Free fluid in abdomen Pleural fluid (right)
Left upper quadrant view (Perisplenic or Left Flank View)	Coronal at left flank	Head	Spleen Diaphragm Left kidney Splenorenal space Lung Spine	Free fluid in abdomen Pleural fluid (left)
Pelvic sagittal view (Retrovesical, Retrouterine, or Pouch of Douglas View)	Sagittal at suprapubic area	Head	Symphysis pubis Bladder Uterus, retro vesical and retroutrine space in females Prostate and retro vesical space in males	Free fluid in abdomen Pregnancy

---

[5] AIUM Practice Parameter for the Performance of the Focused Assessment With Sonography for Trauma (FAST) Examination, © 2014 by the American Institute of Ultrasound in Medicine.

Pelvic transversal view (Retrovesical, Retrouterine, or Pouch of Douglas View)	Transverse at suprapubic area	Right side	Bladder Uterus, retro vesical and retroutrine space in females Prostate and retro vesical space in males	Free fluid in abdomen Pregnancy
Anterior thoracic view	Sagittal at the second intercostal space in the midclavicular line	Head	2 ribs Lung Pleura Chest wall	Pneumothorax

ADDITIONAL VIEWS

View	Site of the probe	Indicator towards Patient's	Visible structures	Expected pathology
Pericolic Gutter Views	Coronal at left flank	Head	Lower pole of the kidney Intestinal loops	Intraperitoneal fluid
The Parasternal View	Sagittal left parasternal space	Head	Heart Lung Spine Aorta	Absent or abnormal cardiac activity Pericardial fluid
The Apical View	At the nipple line at the left fifth intercostal space and aiming it toward the spine or the right shoulder.		Heart Lung	Absent or abnormal cardiac activity Pericardial fluid

SUBXIPHOID VIEW

This view uses the left lobe of the liver as an acoustic window to visualize the heart. The probe is placed transversally at the subxiphoid area with slight angulation towards the left (probe towards the patient's left shoulder). A slight posterior tilt of the probe is helpful to direct the ultrasound beam to the heart. The indicator is towards the patient's right side.

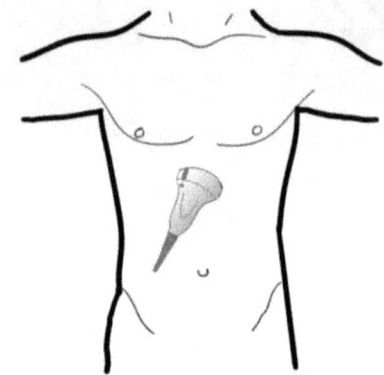

In this view look for:
- Cardiac activity, when absent start reanimation immediately.
- Pericardiac fluid, the nature of the fluid is determined according to the clinical situation. For example, in blunt chest/abdomen trauma it is most likely a hemoperitoneum.

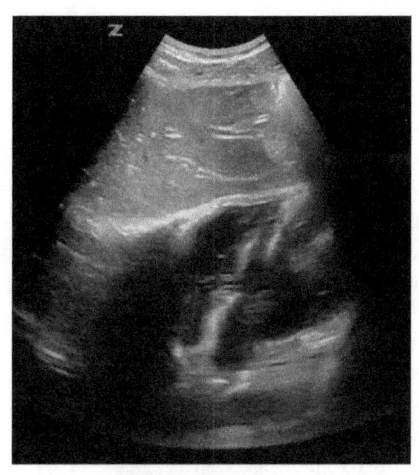

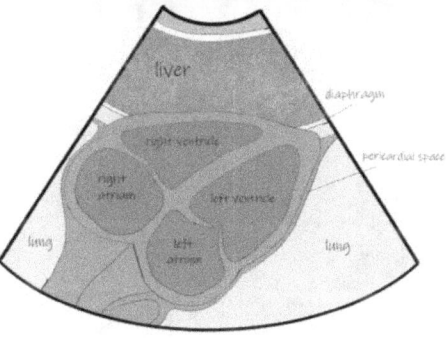

pericardial fluid

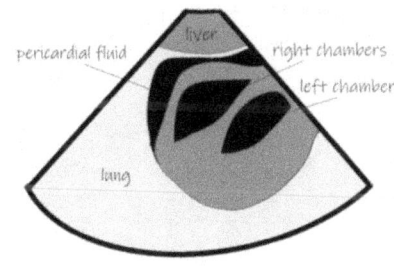

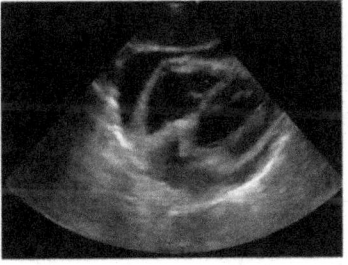

Inferior Vena Cava view

The probe should be placed sagittaly in the subxiphoid area with a slight posterior tilt, so that the beam could be directed towards the patient's right axilla. The indicator is towards the patient's head.

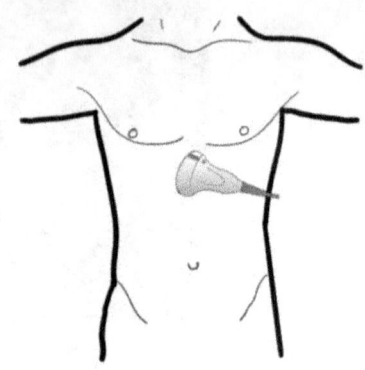

The IVC should be seen passing through the liver. As seen in the picture below, the liver should be seen above and below the IVC. Hepatic veins could be seen entering the IVC. The IVC ends in a wider chamber which is the right atrium.

The physiological slight change in IVC diameter with respiration is a normal finding.

In this view look for:

- Exaggerated change in IVC diameter with respiration until total collapse or what is known as a "Flat IVC" is a sign of hypovolemia. Strat fluid resuscitation.

- Loss of the physiological change in diameter or a distended IVC is a sign of fluid overload. Reconsider the amount of fluid given to the patient.

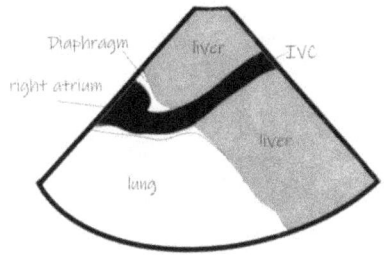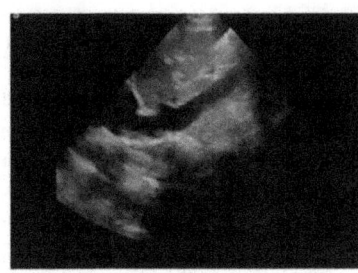

collapsed IVC in Hypovolemia

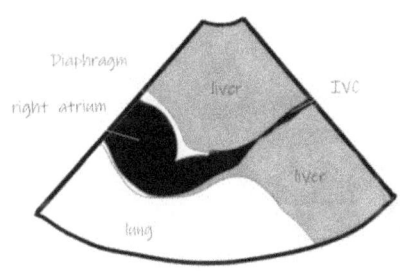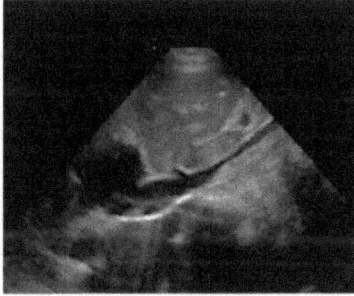

RIGHT UPPER QUADRANT VIEW

With the probe placed coronally over the right lower ribs at the posterior axillary line, start the scan towards the anterior abdominal wall. Then move downwards to scan lower half of the right upper quadrant by moving again backwards towards the posterior axillary line. The indicator is towards the patient's head.

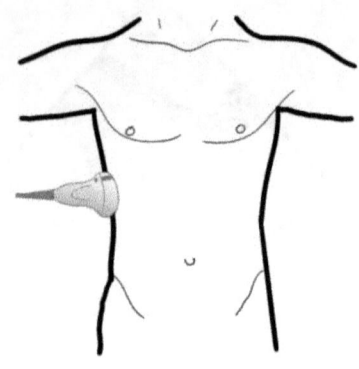

In this view look for

- Free fluid in the abdomen. This can be seen in the hepatorenal (Morison) pouch as a sharp-edged anechoic collection. Don't forget to scan the lower pole of the kidney and the liver dome to exclude the presence of small amounts of free fluid.
- Pleural fluid. The mirroring effect is used to confirm the absence of pleural fluid. Absence of liver mirrored image above the diaphragm, as well as the presence of anechoic area indicates the presence of pleural fluid.

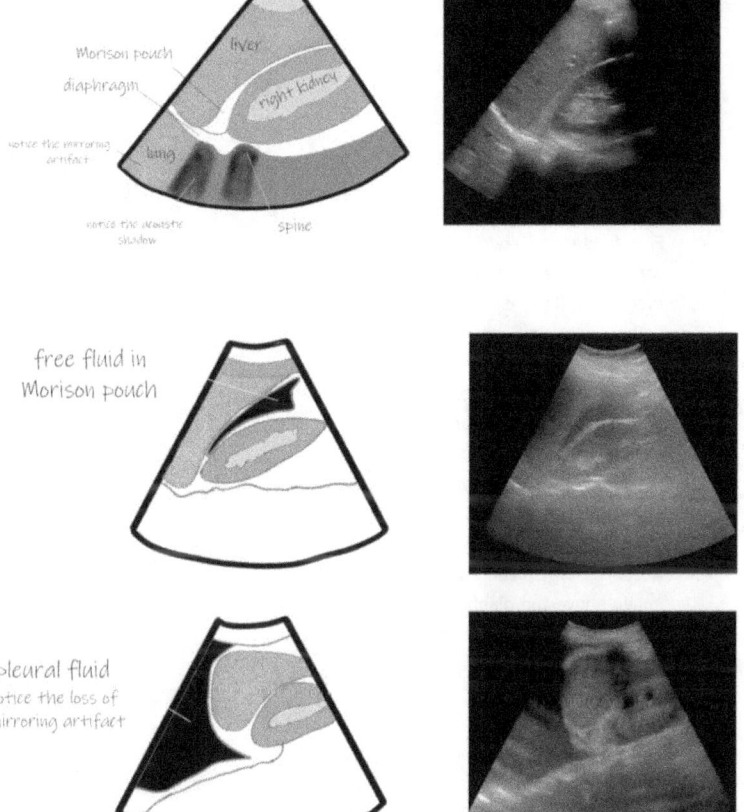

Morison pouch

diaphragm

notice the mirroring artifact

liver

right kidney

lung

notice the acoustic shadow

spine

free fluid in Morison pouch

pleural fluid
notice the loss of mirroring artifact

LEFT UPPER QUADRANT VIEW

With the probe placed coronally over the left lower ribs at the posterior axillary line, start the scan towards the anterior abdominal wall. Then move downwards to scan lower half of the left upper quadrant by moving again backwards towards the posterior axillary line. The indicator is towards the patient's head.

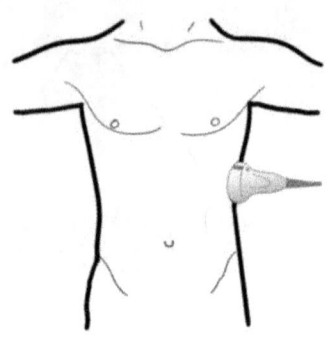

In this view look for

- Free fluid in the abdomen. This can be seen around the spleen more than in the splenorenal pouch as a sharp-edged anechoic collection. Don't forget to scan the lower pole of the kidney to exclude the presence of small amounts of free fluid.

- Pleural fluid. The mirroring effect is used to confirm the absence of pleural fluid. Absence of spleen mirrored image above the diaphragm, as well as the presence of anechoic area indicates the presence of pleural fluid.

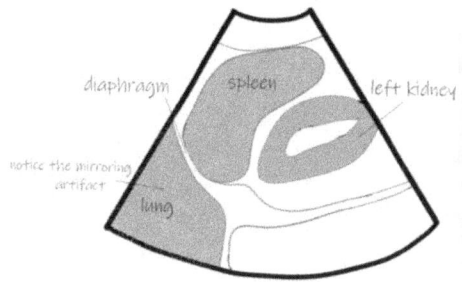
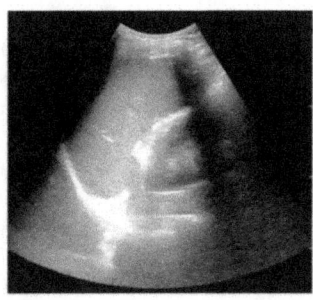

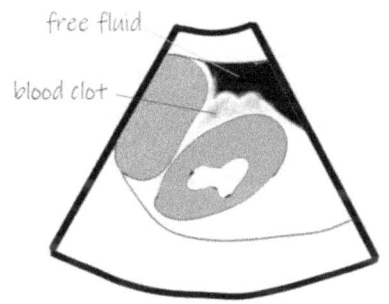
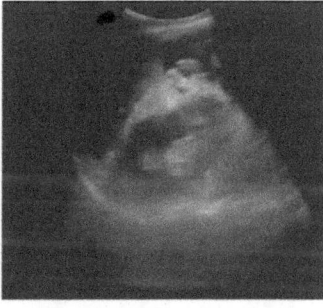

PELVIC SAGITTAL VIEW

Strat the scan by placing the probe sagittaly in the suprapubic area. The indicator is towards the patient's head. The symphysis pubis is identified at lower end of the image by it acoustic shadow. A full bladder is useful as an acoustic window. When necessary the bladder can be filled either by clamping the Foley catheter or by injecting fluid in it.

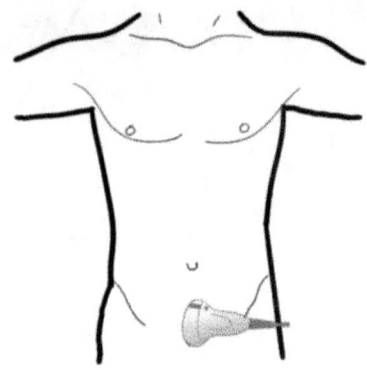

In this view look for

- Free fluid in the abdomen tends to accumulate in the most dependent area which is the pelvis. In this view look for fluid in male patients above the urinary bladder in the intraperitoneal space. While in female patients, fluid can also accumulate between the bladder and the uterus in the Douglas pouch
- Pregnancy.

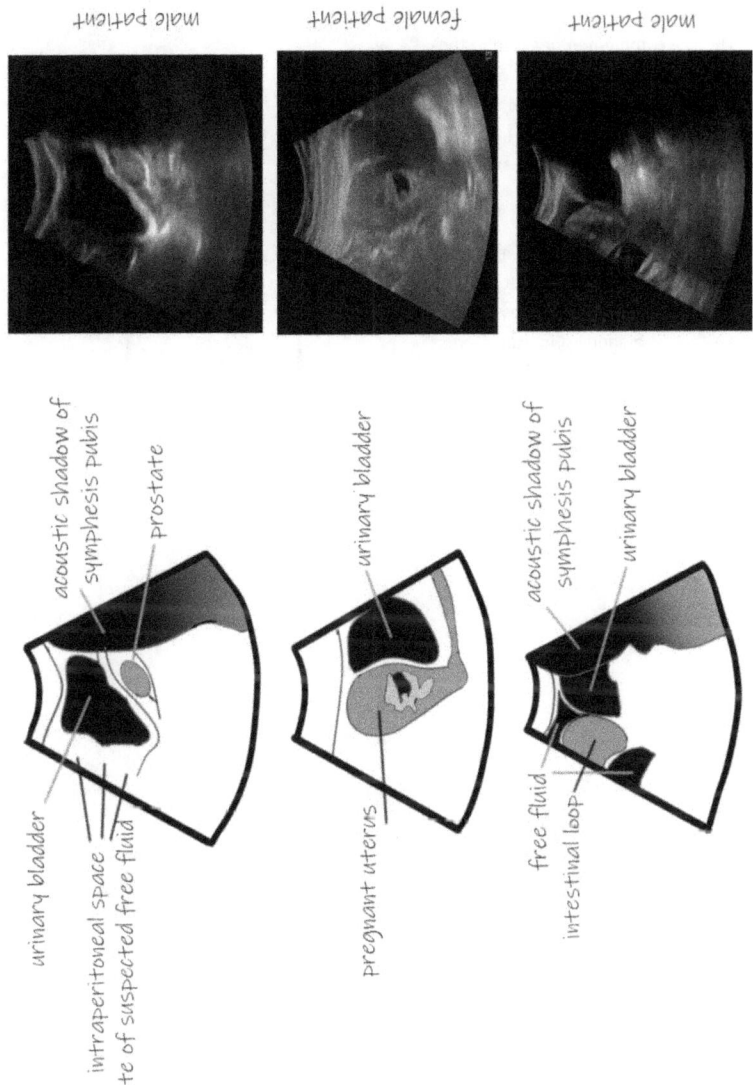

male patient

Female patient

male patient

acoustic shadow of symphesis pubis

prostate

urinary bladder

urinary bladder

intraperitoneal space

site of suspected free fluid

pregnant uterus

acoustic shadow of symphesis pubis

urinary bladder

free fluid

intestinal loop

PELVIC TRANSVERSAL VIEW

This is a complementary scan to the previous pelvic view. The probe is placed transversally in the suprapubic area with the indicator towards the patient's right side.

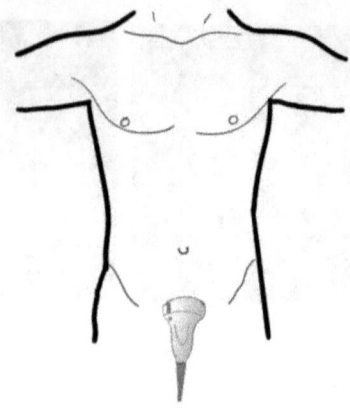

In this view look for
- Free fluid in the abdomen especially in the lateral sides of the bladder and the uterus which couldn't be thoroughly evaluated in the pelvic sagittal view.
- Pregnancy.

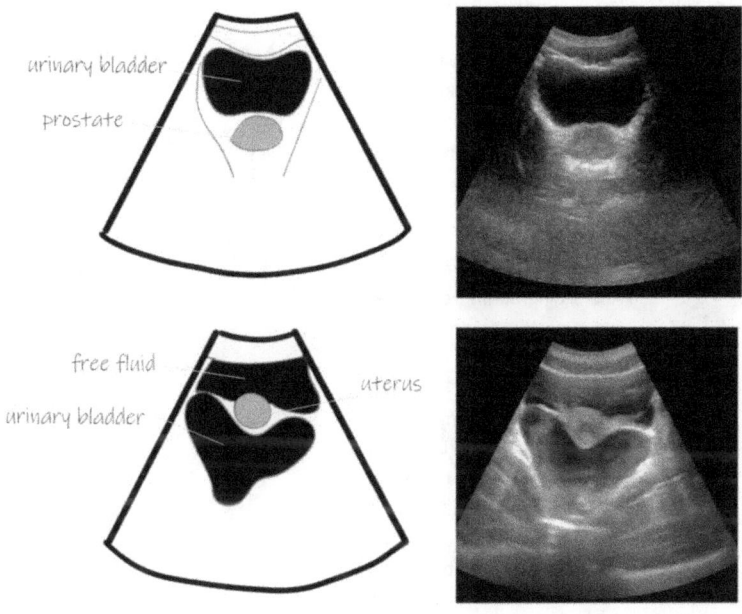

urinary bladder
prostate

free fluid
urinary bladder
uterus

ANTERIOR THORACIC VIEW

This view is dedicated to the detection of pneumothorax. The probe could be placed sagittaly between any 2 rips at the midclavicular line, but typically the second or third intercostal spaces are used. The indicator is towards the patient's head. Only the pleural line sliding movement is evaluated in the near field, so a superficial probe may be used as well.

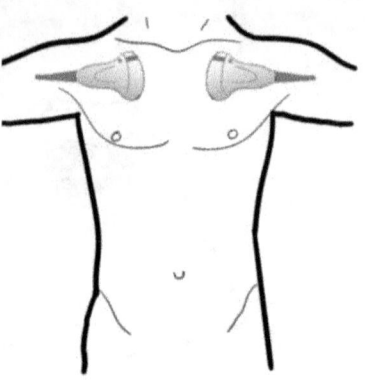

In this view look for

- Absence the normal pleural line sliding during respiration indicates the presence of air between the parietal and visceral pleura (Pneumothorax). This sliding movement should be easily recognized in the normal B mode. If not move to the M mode.

- The M mode is plotting each point in a certain vertical line against time (transverse axis). Static or not moving structures will show a clear flat line, while moving structures will be plotted as hazy area as shown below. Look for the normal appearance of the sea shore sign that indicates normal pleural sliding movement.

B mode

second rib   third rib notice the acoustic shadows

lung

pleura

thoracic wall

second intercostal space

pleural line sliding with respiration indicates normal lung ventilation in absence of pneumothorax

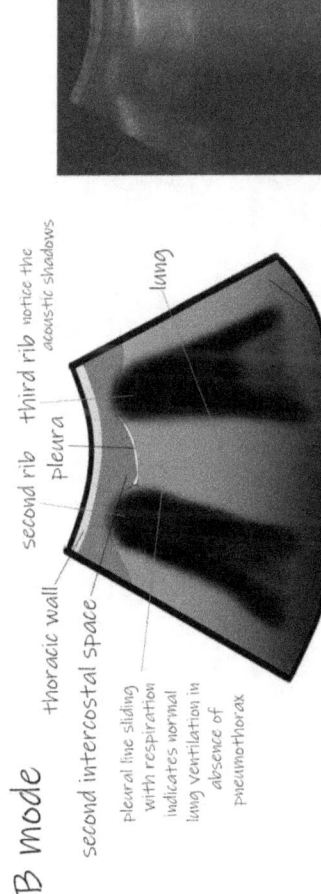

M mode

the not moving thoracic wall appears as continuous lines. On the other hand the sliding movement of the lung appears as a hazy or texture area

thoracic wall
pleura
lung

normal lung
sea shore sign

pneumothorax

both thoracic wall and lung underneath are not moving due to pneumothorax. both appears as continuous lines.

thoracic wall
pleura
lung

CHAPTER 8

ECG

Contents

Introduction and basic concepts   135
ECG waves, segments and intervals   142
ECG changes with common cardiological conditions   150
Heart chambers hypertrophy or dilation   150
Myocardial ischemia   152
Myocardial infarction   154
Electrolyte disturbances   156
Heart block   157
Arrhythmia   159
How to write ECG report   163

INTRODUCTION AND BASICS CONCEPTS

✓ ECG is an easy method of recording the electrical activity of the heart. It demonstrates the relationship between the direction of electrical activity, the current amplitude and the duration of this electrical activity.

✓ An ECG gives two types of data:

- It clarifies how long a stimulation wave or action potential wave takes to travel from one part of the heart to the next and so it clarifies if the electrical activity is normal, slow, fast, regular or irregular.

- It measures the strength or amplitude of electrical activity which travels through the heart.

✓ Interpretation of the ECG helps us to reach the right diagnosis. So, we can say that ECG interpretation itself is not a Diagnosis.

✓ Here, in this chapter we will discuss shortly how we can use this magnificent tool (ECG) and so we must answer three main questions.

- The first question is: How to comment on ECG?

- The second question is: What is the deferential diagnosis of ECG waves abnormalities?

- The third question is: How can the ECG helps in diagnosis of arrhythmias, myocardial hypoperfusion and electrolyte disorders?

NORMAL MORPHOLOGY OF ECG

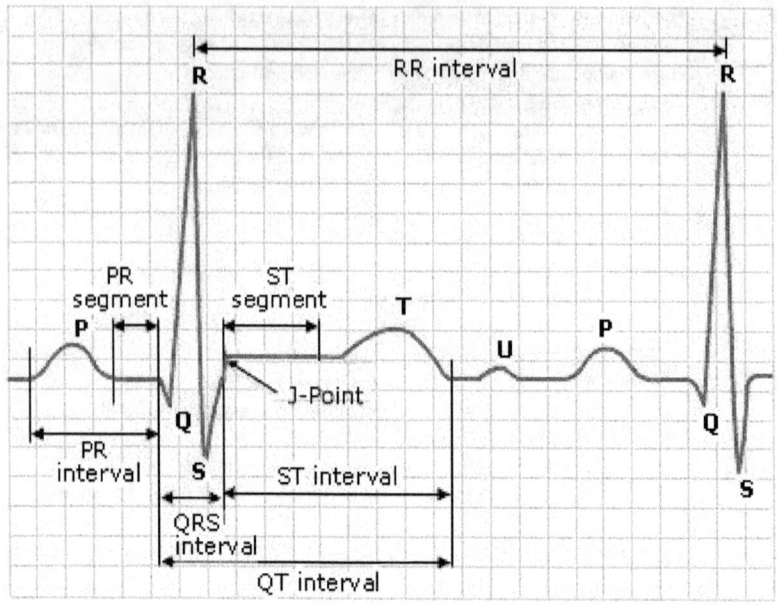

ECG GRID AND HEART RATE CALCULATION

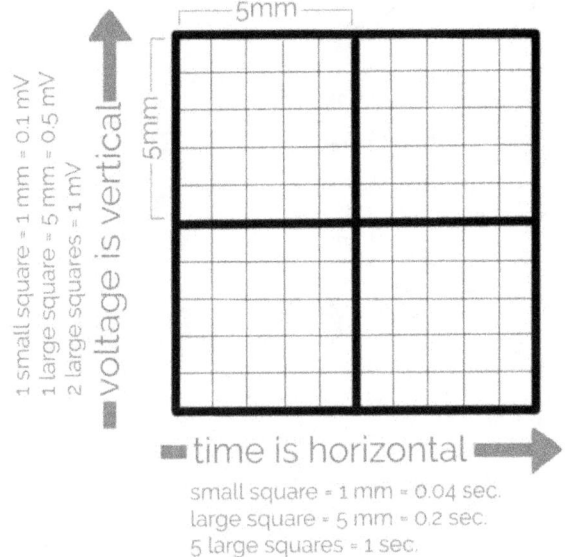

small square = 1 mm = 0.04 sec.
large square = 5 mm = 0.2 sec.
5 large squares = 1 sec.

There are several ways to calculate the heart rate based on ECG. While the device always gives you the heart rate in the hand, it is always wise to double check.

METHOD #1: THE RR INTERVAL.

Count the large squares in one RR interval (the interval between 2 consecutive R waves) and then refer to the table below for the quick reference. This method is only valid for regular rhythm.

Large squares in 1 RR interval	1	2	3	4	5	6	7	8
Beats per minute	300	150	100	75	60	50	43	37

METHOD #2: COUNTING THE R WAVES

Count the R waves in 50 large squares (10 sec.) and then multiply result times 6 to get the heart rate in one minute. This gives a better estimation in cases showing irregular rhythm.

12 LEADS ECG

Group	Lead	Position	Normal wave
Lateral leads — Looking at the heart through lateral wall of the left ventricle	I	+ve: left arm -ve: right arm	
	aVL	Left arm	
	V5	Same as V4 at left anterior axillary line	
	V6	Same as V4 at left midaxillary line	
Anterior leads — Looking at the anterior wall of both ventricles	V3	Midway between V2 and V4	
	V4	5th intercostal space midclavicular line	
Septal leads — Looking at the interventricular septum	V1	4th intercostal space right to the sternum	
	V2	4th intercostal space left to the sternum	
Inferior leads — Looking at the inferior (diaphragmatic) surface of the heart	II	+ve: left leg -ve: right arm	
	III	+ve: left leg -ve: left arm	
	aVF	Left leg	
	aVR	Left arm	

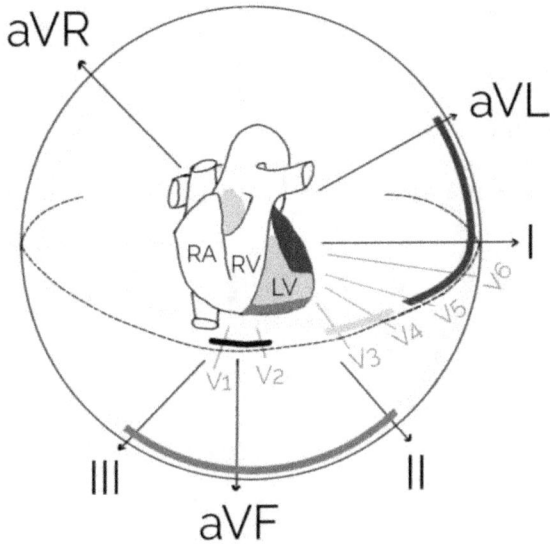

DIRECTION OF THE WAVES IN DIFFERENT LEADS

If the depolarisation wave is in the same direction of the lead, the graph created will be a positive (upwards) wave and vice versa. This means that opposite leads (e.g. Lead II and aVR) are mirror images of each other.

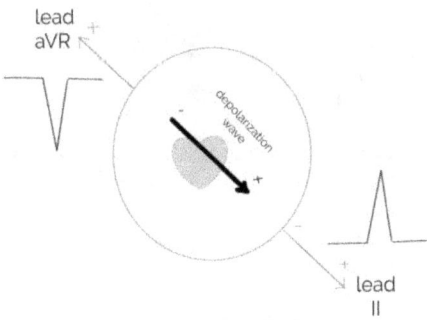

THE CARDIAC AXIS

Cardiac Axis is the summation of the overall depolarization waves of the heart.

Types of Cardiac Axis:

- Normal Axis
- Left Axis Deviation.
- Right Axis Deviation.
- Extreme Axis Deviation.

Cardiac Axis is determined by evaluation of the QRS Complex in Leads I, II and III as in the table below.

Leads	Normal Axis	Left Axis Deviation	Right Axis Deviation	Extreme Axis Deviation
QRS in lead I	+ ve	+ve	-ve	-ve
QRS in lead II	+ve	-ve	+ve	-ve
QRS in lead III	+ve	-ve	+ve	-ve

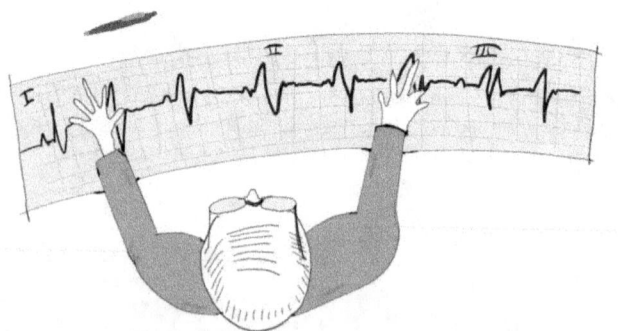

A simple way to this is by putting your left hand on Lead I and your right hand on lead III as you read the ECG strip and examine the QRS complexes.

- ✓ If they are positive (upwards) in all leads, then it is a positive point; there is no axis deviation.
- ✓ If they are negative (downwards) in all leads, then this a very negative result; an extreme axis deviation.
- ✓ If they are different from each other, then the axis is deviated towards the hand on the positive lead. i.e. Lead I is positive (with your left hand on it), then it is a left axis deviation, and vice versa.

MOST COMMON CAUSES OF CARDIAC AXIS DEVIATION:[6]

Left axis deviation	Right axis deviation
Normal variant (physiologic, age-related)	Normal variant (physiologic, age-related)
Congenital heart disease (eg. Primum ASD)	Congenital heart disease (e.g., secundum ASD)
Emphysema	Left pneumothorax
Left ventricular hypertrophy	Right ventricular overload, Right ventricular hypertrophy
Inferior wall myocardial infarction (acute onset)	Lateral wall myocardial infarction. (acute onset)
left bundle branch block.	Right bundle branch block
left anterior fascicular block.	Left posterior fascicular block,
Atrioventricular re-entry Tachycardia (e.g., Wolff-Parkinson-White syndrome)	Atrioventricular re-entry Tachycardia (e.g., Wolff-Parkinson-White syndrome)
ventricular tachycardia	Ventricular tachycardia.
Hyperkalaemia.	Dextrocardia
Mechanical: deep expiration or elevated diaphragm (e.g. abdominal masses, organomegaly, ascites and pregnancy)	Mechanical: deep inspiration or emphysema
	Conditions that cause right-ventricular strain (e.g., pulmonary embolism, pulmonary stenosis, pulmonary hypertension, chronic lung disease, and resultant cor pulmonale)

[6] Kashou AH, Kashou HE. Electrical Axis (Normal, Right Axis Deviation, and Left Axis Deviation) [Updated 2018 Oct 27]. In: StatPearls [Internet]. Treasure Island (FL): StatPearls Publishing; 2019 Jan-. Available from: https://www.ncbi.nlm.nih.gov/books/NBK470532/

ECG WAVES, SEGMENTS AND INTERVALS

MORPHOLOGY AND COMMON PATHOLOGICAL FINDINGS

P WAVE

Amplitude: <0.2 mV

Duration: 50-100 ms

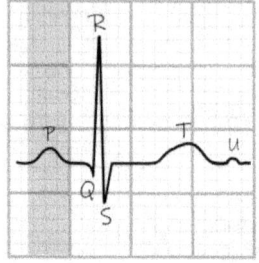

Common Pathological findings

- Absent P wave:
    - Atrial Fibrillation
    - AV Rhythm (P wave is masked with QRS complex)
- ↑ Amplitude: (P Pulmonal)
    - Young adults.
    - Right Atrial dilatation.
    - Cor pulmonal, COPD, Chronic Bronchitis.
    - Pulmonary stenosis, Tricuspid regurgitation.
- ↑ Duration or bifid P wave: (P Mitral) Left Atrial dilatation.
    - Mitral valve lesions (Stenosis or regurgitation)
    - Aortic valve lesions (Stenosis or regurgitation)
    - PDA
    - Hypertension
    - Constrictive pericarditis
- Inverted P wave:
    - o ectopic pacemaker cells in atria.
    - o retrograde stimulation.
    - o AV Block

Q WAVE

Amplitude: Q wave normally is less than 15% of the
R wave amplitude.

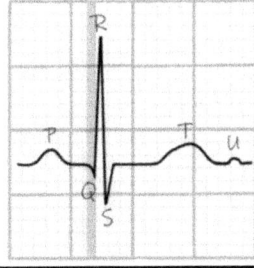

Common abnormal findings

Deep Q wave ≥ 25% of the amplitude of R wave

- o Myocardial infarction, (deep Q wave is a sign of established transmural <u>death</u> of myocardium which is called "Electrical window").
- o Normal variant.
- o Right ventricular hypertrophy +/- RBBB
- o Hyperkalaemia
- o Acute pancreatitis
- o WPW syndrome
- o false positioning of ECG electrodes.
- o Left side Pneumothorax.

QRS Complex

Amplitude: Less than 3 mV

Duration: 60-100 ms.

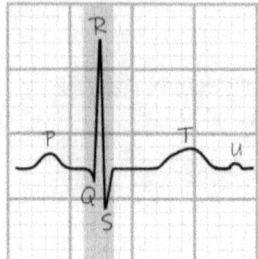

Common abnormal findings

Amplitude of QRS complex is algebraic summation of R and S waves.

Large QRS Complex:
- o Young Adult or normal variation.
- o Fever
- o Hyperthyroidism
- o Anaemia
- o **Left side hypertrophy:**
  Tall R wave in V_5 and deep S wave V_1

  Sokolow Lyon Index for left ventricular hypertrophy:

  R wave in V_5 + S wave in $V_1 \geq 3.5$ Mv

- o **Right side hypertrophy:**
  R wave in V_1 and potentially deep S wave in V_5

  Sokolow Lyon Index for right ventricular hypertrophy:

  S wave in V_5 + R wave in $V_1 \geq 1.05$ mV

Low voltage small QRS complex:
- o Normal variation
- o Obesity.
- o Pregnancy.
- o COPD.
- o Pleural effusion.
- o Myocardial effusion.
- o Myocarditis
- o Hypothyroidism
- o Ischemia.
- o Cardiomyopathy
- o Myocardial Infiltration

Narrow QRS Complex:
- o Sinus Tachycardia.
- o Supraventricular tachycardia.
- o Atrial flatter
- o Tachyarrhythmia on top of Atrial fibrillation.

Broad QRS Complex:
- o Ventricular Extrasystole
- o Left Bundle Branch Block (complete or incomplete) LBBB
- o Right Bundle Branch Block (complete or incomplete) RBBB
- o Ventricular Tachycardia (VT)
- o WPW syndrome.

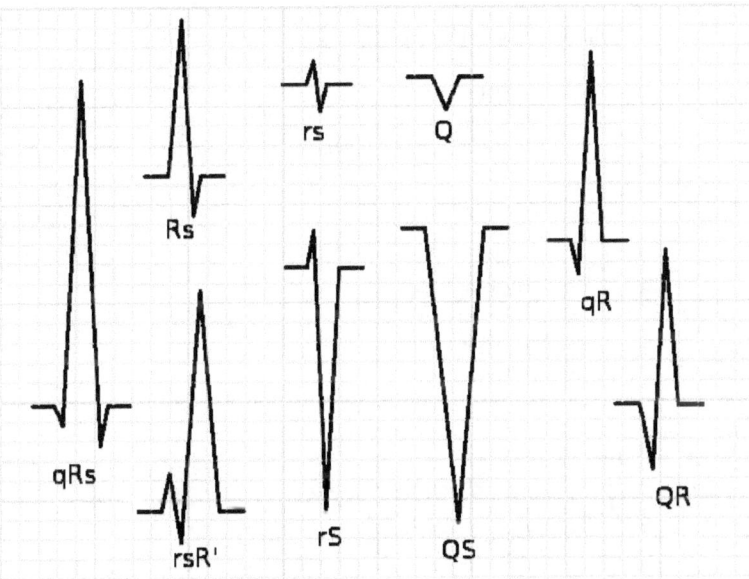

Variable nomenclature of the QRS complex based on the form of the waves, note that the high amplitude waves are assigned uppercase letters, while the low amplitude waves are assigned lowercase letters.

T WAVE

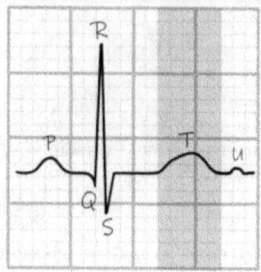

Common abnormal findings

Peaked T wave: T wave is more than 2/3 the amplitude of R wave.

- o Ischemic Causes: (Hyperacute T wave)
    - Acute sever myocardial Hypoperfusion (unstable angina)
    - Posterior wall infraction (chest leads V 2-5)
    - Initial phase of the anterior wall infraction (chest leads V 2-5)
- o Non-ischemic causes:
    - Adult.
    - Athletics.
    - Hyperkalaemia.
    - Hemopericardium.
    - Left side strain.
    - LBBB.

Flat T wave:
- o Hypokalaemia
- o Hypoaldosteronism (Addison disease)
- o Hypothyroidism
- o Hypoperfusion (Myocardial Ischemia) CAD
- o Pericardial effusion

Inverted T wave:
- o Normal variant
- o Myocardial ischemia, Infraction
- o Digitalis toxicity
- o Cerebro-vascular accidents.
- o Toxicity
- o Left ventricular hypertrophy.

U WAVE

Abnormal wave

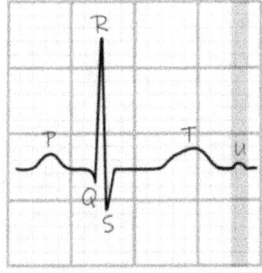

Common abnormal findings
o   Athletics.
o   Excessive vagal stimulation.
o   Hypokalaemia.
o   Hypothyroidism.

PR INTERVAL

Normal Duration of PR Interval is: 0.12 - 0.20 ms.

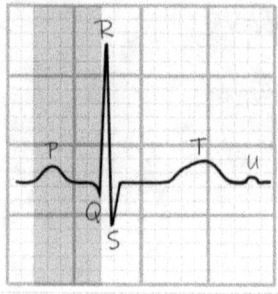

Common abnormal findings

Long PR:

- o Increased vagal Tone.
- o AV Block.
- o Myocardial Ischemia.
- o Drugs.
- o Hypothyroidism.
- o Myocarditis / Endocarditis.
- o Hypothermia.

Short PR:

- o Tachycardia.
- o Hyperthyroidism.
- o WPW or LGL Syndrome.
- o Ectopic atrial stimulating focus or external pacemaker.

ST SEGMENT

Normally isoelectric.

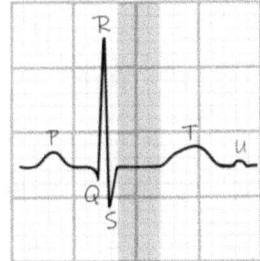

Common abnormal findings

ST Elevation:
- o   STEMI: ST Elevation Myocardial Infraction (elevation > 0.2mV)
- o   Transmural Ischemia.
- o   Left side ventricular strain.
- o   Excessive vagal tone.
- o   Pulmonary embolism.

ST Depression:
- o   Myocardial ischemia (CAD)
- o   Left side hypertrophy or myocardial strain (e.g. Systemic Hypertension, Aortic valve lesions)
- o   Posterior wall Infraction.
- o   LBBB.
- o   Hypokalaemia.
- o   Cardiomyopathy.
- o   Digitalis toxicity.
- o   CO toxicity.
- o   Antiarrhythmic drugs.
- o   SLE.
- o   Rheumatoid arthritis.

ECG CHANGES WITH COMMON CARDIOLOGICAL CONDITIONS

HEART CHAMBERS HYPERTROPHY OR DILATION

LEFT ATRIAL ENLARGEMENT:
P mitral: Broad notched or Bifid P wave and longer than 0.12 sec.

RIGHT ATRIAL ENLARGEMENT:
P pulmonal: Peaked p wave i.e. taller than 3 mm or 0.3 mV.

	Lead II	Lead V2
Left atrial hypertrophy (P mitrale)	Broad and notched (> 0.12)	Inverted
Right atrial hypertrophy (P pulmonale)	Peaked (>3mm)	Upright
Combined atrial hypertrophy	May be both peaked and broad	Biphasic ("peaked" and "Broad")

Left ventricular hypertrophy:
Sokolov-Lyon criteria (S wave depth in V1 + tallest R wave height in V5-V6 > 35 mm)

Left ventricular strain:
ST depression and T wave inversion in the lateral leads.

Right ventricular hypertrophy:
Predominant R wave in V1 - Predominant S wave in V5 or V6
Sokolow Lyon Index right ventricle: The sum of the voltage of R wave in Lead V2 and the S wave in lead V5 is more than 1.1 mV. R (V2) + S (V5) > 1.1 mV.

Right ventricular strain e.g. Pulmonary Embolism:
right axis deviation, S1 Q3 T3 and T-wave inversions in V1-4 and lead III.

MYOCARDIAL ISCHEMIA[7]

Suspected Changes:

1- **ST depression:**
   Forms: can be either upsloping, down sloping, or horizontal.

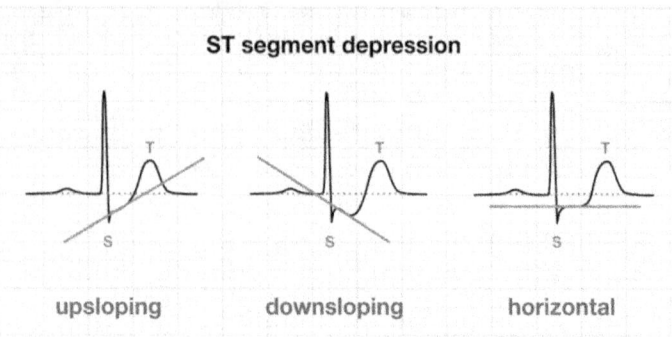

ST segment depression

upsloping   downsloping   horizontal

- o   Horizontal or down sloping ST depression ≥ 0.5 mm at the J-point in ≥ 2 contiguous leads indicates myocardial ischaemia.
- o   ST depression ≥ 1 mm is more specific and predicts bad prognosis.
- o   ST depression ≥ 2 mm in ≥ 3 leads is accompanied with a high probability of NSTEMI.
- o   Upsloping ST depression is non-specific for myocardial ischaemia.

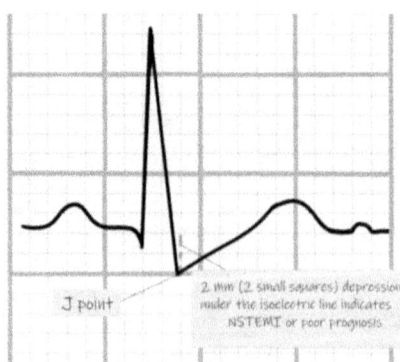

J point

2 mm (2 small squares) depression under the isoelectric line indicates NSTEMI or poor prognosis

2- **T wave inversion:**

---

[7] European Heart Journal, Volume 39, Issue 2, 07 January 2018, Pages 119–177

- can considered as evidence of myocardial ischemia in the following conditions:
- If recently occurred T wave inversion.
- Deeper than 1mm (0.1 mV)
- Present in more than 2 leads in which presents predominant R wave. (i.e R/S ratio > 1)

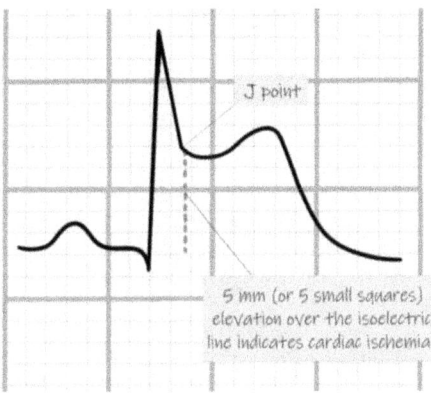

J point

5 mm (or 5 small squares) elevation over the isoelectric line indicates cardiac ischemia

Myocardial Infraction

ECG CHANGES IN THE DIFFERENT STAGES OF MYOCARDIAL INFRACTION[8]

Stage	Changes
Early stage: (minutes after coronary artery occlusion)	Tall peaked Hyperacute T wave
Stage I: (in the first 6 hours)	ST segment elevation +/- small Q wave
Intermediate stage (after 6 hours)	ST segment elevation T wave inversion Pathological Q wave (mostly after 12 hours)
Stage II (2-4 weeks up to months)	Prominent Q wave. ST segment normalisation (>2 weeks in inferior MI, >4 weeks in anterior MI) Inverted T wave.
Stage III (end stage or old MI)	Persistent Q wave Normal ST segment, or may be accompanied with ST depression due to remaining other ischemic manifestations. NB. Persistent ST elevation is suggesting for occurrence of myocardial aneurysm.

ST ELEVATION MYOCARDIAL INFRACTION (STEMI)[9]
- ST-segment elevation in two contiguous leads ≥ 2.5 mm in men less than 40 years.
- ST-segment elevation in two contiguous leads ≥2 mm in men older than 40 years.
- ST-segment elevation in two contiguous leads ≥ 1.5 mm in women in leads (V2, V3) and/or greater than 1 mm in the other leads.

NON-ST ELEVATION MYOCARDIAL INFARCTION (NSTEMI):
- Chest pain and positive serum troponin I level.
- there are no characteristic ECG changes (may be only ischemic picture)

---

[8] ABC of clinical electrocardiography, Francis Morris and William J Brady, BMJ. 2002 Apr 6; 324(7341): 831–834.

[9] European Heart Journal, Volume 39, Issue 2, 07 January 2018, Pages 119–177

LOCALISATION OF MYOCARDIAL INFRACTION[10]

Left main coronary artery	Left Anterior Descending coronary artery	Anterior MI	ST elevation in Leads V1 to V4
		Lateral MI	Leads I, aVL, V5, and V6.
		Septal MI	ST elevation in Leads V1 to V2-3
	Circumflex coronary artery	Lateral MI	Leads I, aVL, V5, and V6
		Posterior MI	ST elevation in leads V7 to V9 (over the posterior chest wall) ST depression in V1, V2, V3 Prominent R wave in V1, V2, V3
		Postero-lateral MI	ST elevation in leads V7 to V9, I, aVL, V5, and V6. ST depression in V1, V2, V3
		Infero-posterior MI	ST elevation in leads: II, III, aVF, V7, V8, V9 ST depression, prominent R wave and prominent T wave in leads: V1, V2 and V3
Right main coronary artery		Inferior wall:	ST elevation: Leads II, III, and aVF. ST depression: leads aVL
		Posterior wall	ST elevation: Leads V7 to V9 (over the posterior chest wall) ST depression, prominent R wave and prominent T wave in leads: V1, V2 and V3
		Infero-lateral MI	ST elevation: II, III, aVF, aVL, V5, V6, V4r
		Infero-posterior	ST elevation: II, III, aVF, V7, V8, V9. ST depression, prominent R wave and prominent T wave in leads: V1, V2 and V3.
		Inferior MI with right ventricular MI	ST elevation: II, III, aVF, V4r, V1, V2.

[10] Electrocardiographic Localization of Coronary Artery Narrowings: Studies During Myocardial Ischemia and Infarction in Patients with One-vessel Disease, RICHARD M. FUCHS, M.D., STEPHEN C. ACHUFF, M.D., LouISE GRUNWALD, B.A. et al., Circulation. 1982 Dec;66(6):1168-76.

ELECTROLYTE DISTURBANCES

Hyperkalemia	Tall peaked T waves. Broad QRS complexes, RBBB, LBBB and tri-fascicular block till development of Development of a sine wave pattern. P wave changes (progressive decrease in P wave amplitude).
Hypokalemia	ST segment depression. Decreased T wave amplitude. Prominent U wave. Different types of arrhythmias Prolonged QRS duration. increased P wave amplitude and duration
Hypercalcemia	Short Q-T interval
Hypocalcemia	Prolonged Q-T interval
Hypomagnesaemia	Flat T waves. ST segment depression. prominent U waves. prolonged P-R interval.
Hypermagnesaemia	prolonged P-R interval. wide QRS complexes.

Heart Block

First-Degree AV block: prolonged PR interval > 0.2 s

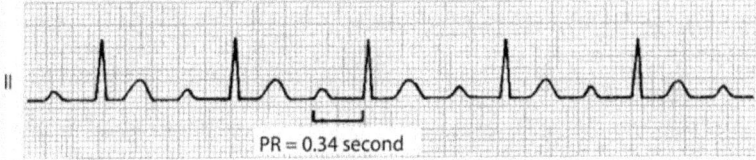

PR = 0.34 second

Second-Degree AV Block Type I - Mobitz I (Wenkebach): progressive PR interval prolongation until a P wave is not followed with QRS complex. -irregular R-R interval.

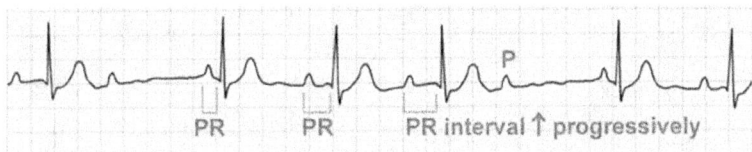

PR   PR   PR interval ↑ progressively

Second-Degree AV Block Type II - Mobitz II:
-There are dropped QRS complex without PR interval prolongation.
-the rate of P waves: QRS complexes is fixed and may be 2:1, 3:1, 4:1.
-Some P waves are not followed by QRS complex.
-PR interval (if the beat is conducted) beats will be constant across the strip.

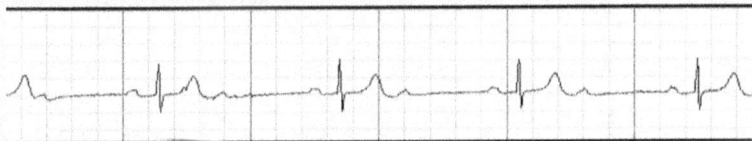

Third degree AV Block:
-There is complete dissociation between atrial and ventricular rhythm.
-P-P and R-R intervals are regular.
-PR interval is irregular, and there is no relation between P wave and QRS complex.

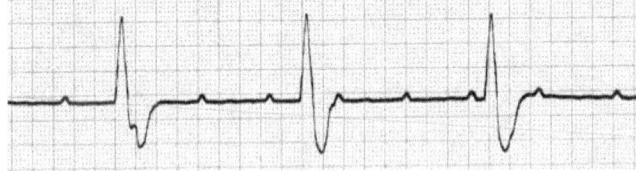

Right bundle branch block (RBBB)
-QRS duration >0.12 seconds.
-Right axis deviation.
-Slurred S wave in lead I, aVL, V5, and V6.
-RSR' in V1 and V2.

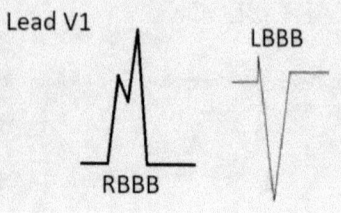

Left bundle branch block (LBBB)
-QRS duration >0.12 seconds.
-Left axis deviation.
-Broad R waves in I, aVL, V5, and V6.
-Broad, dominant S wave in V1 and V2.
-RSR' in V5 and V6.

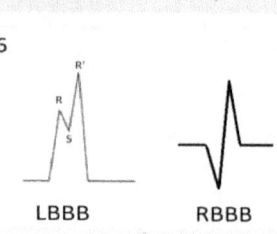

Left anterior fascicular block (LAFB)
-Prolonged QRS duration.
-Left axis deviation
-qR complex in leads I and aVL.
-rS complex in leads II, III, and aVF.

Left Posterior Fascicular Block (LPFB)
-Slightly prolonged QRS duration.
-Right axis deviation
-qR complex in leads II, III, and aVF.
-rS complex in leads I and aVL.

Bifascicular Block
-It is the combination of RBBB with either LAFB or LPFB.
-most commonly RBBB + LAFB = RBBB findings + left axis deviation

Trifascicular Block
Complete trifascicular block
Bifascicular block + 3rd degree AV block
Incomplete trifascicular block
Bifascicular block + 1st degree AV block (most common)
Bifascicular block + 2nd degree AV block
RBBB + alternating LAFB / LPFB

ARRHYTHMIA

SINUS ARRHYTHMIAS

Respiratory sinus arrhythmia
Physiological changes in the R-R interval during respiration: reduced during inspiration (Tachycardia) and increase during expiration (Bradycardia)

Loss of respiratory sinus arrhythmia
No or minimal changes in R-R interval during inspiration (DD: advanced DM, old age and digitalis toxicity)

Sinus Tachycardia
Heart rate up to 180 bpm, regular and accompanied with normal P wave
Gradual onset and offset,

Sinus bradycardia
Heart rate is less than 60 bpm accompanied with normal P wave a normal P-R interval.

Sinoatrial pause or arrest
Sudden and transient disappearance of P wave

Tachycardia –Bradycardia Syndrome (Tachy – Brady- Syndrome)
Intermittent sinus tachycardia and bradycardia as a start for sick sinus syndrome.

SUPRAVENTRICULAR ARRHYTHMIAS

Supraventricular premature beats (Atrial extrasystole)
Abnormal P wave followed with normal QRS complex then there is compensatory pause.
QRS complex: narrow

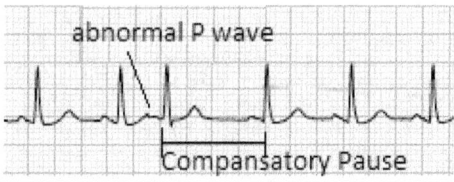

Atrial flutter
Rhythm: regular
Rate: atrial rate between 250–350; ventricular rate is around 150-200
P wave: Sawtooth appearance (flutter waves), more prominent in leads II, III, and aVF
Onset: abrubt
QRS complex: narrow

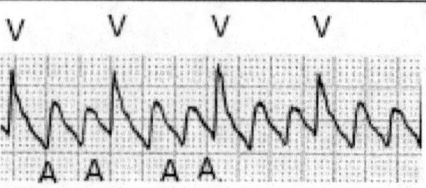

Atrial fibrillation

Rhythm: Irregularly irregularity

Rate: atrial rate between 250–350; ventricular rate is around 150-250

P wave: Absent P wave (only irregular line)

QRS complex: narrow

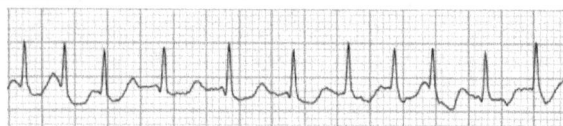

Atrial tachycardia
Focal atrial tachycardia

Rhythm: regular

Rate: atrial rate between 150–250; ventricular rate is around 200

P wave: Different morphology than the original sinus P wave but also single morphological variant (single focus)

Onset: abrubt

QRS complex: narrow

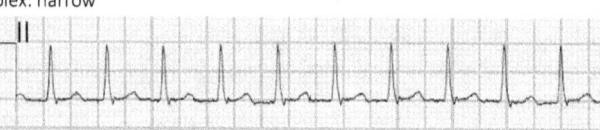

Multifocal atrial tachycardia (MAT)

Rhythm: irregular

Rate: atrial rate between 150–250; ventricular rate is around 200

P wave: Multiple different morphology (more than 3 morphological variants) than the original sinus P wave. (multi-focal origin)

Onset: abrupt

QRS complex: narrow

AV Node Arrhythmias

Atrioventricular reentry Tachycardia (AVRT) Eg. WPW Syndrome.	Rhythm: regular Rate: between 150–250 bpm; P wave: Inverted, and may occur after QRS complex. Onset: abrupt QRS complex: Narrow if orthodromic AVRT Broad (delta wave) if antidromic AVRT

Orthodromic	Antidromic
- common. - Narrow QRS. - Pathology: Forward conduction (from the atrium to the ventricle) pass through the AV node, and retrograde conduction (from ventricle to atrium) pass through the accessory pathway- bundle of Kent.	- rare. - Broad QRS (Delta wave). - Pathology: Forward conduction (from the atrium to the ventricle) pass through the accessory pathway- bundle of Kent, and retrograde conduction (from ventricle to atrium) pass through the the AV node.

Junctional tachycardia	Rhythm: regular Rate: between 100-150 bpm; P wave: Inverted, and may occur before, within or after the QRS complex. Onset: gradual QRS complex: Narrow

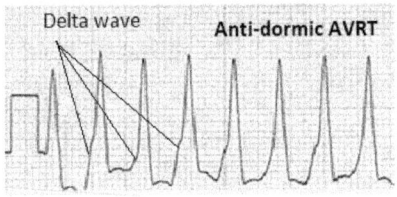

Delta wave   **Anti-dormic AVRT**

Premature ventricular beat (Ventricular extrasystole)
Abnormal wide, early QRS complex which is not preceded by P wave,
and followed with compensatory pause.

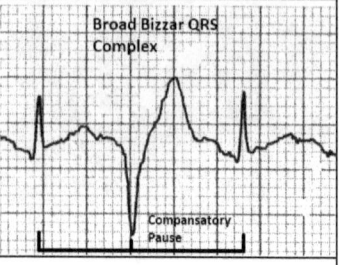

Ventricular tachycardia
Rhythm: regular
Rate: between 80 -150 bpm.
P wave: most commonly absent P wave.
Onset: gradual
QRS complex: more than three successive broad, monomorphic (if single ventricular stimulating focus) or polymorphic (if multiple ventricular stimulating foci)
NB. Torsade de pointes tachycardia: is a form of poly morphic VT (sine wave appearance)

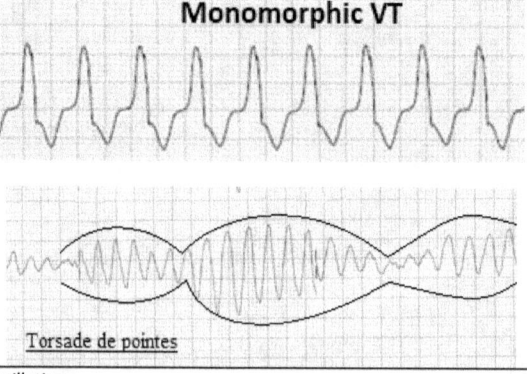

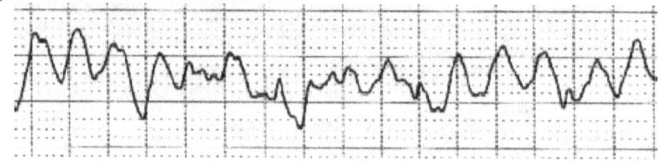

Ventricular fibrillation
Irregular fine fibrillation waves rate > 300.

HOW TO WRITE ECG REPORT?

Personal Data:	Name:			
	Age:	Sex:		Ward:
	Short Diagnosis and clinical details:			
	Drugs:			
Heart Rate:	.... Normal b/m	Tachycardia > 90 beat/min	Bradycardia < 50 beat/min	
Regularity:	Regular	Regular irregularity	Irregular irregularity	
Axis	Normal:	Left axis deviation:	Right axis deviation:	
P wave	Present in I, II, III and followed regularly with R wave → Sinus Rhythm	Present but followed with irregular R wave → II, III-degree HB	Absent: AF Saw teeth: At. Flatter P pulmonal P mitral	
PQ Interval	Normal: 0,12 – 0.2 sec.	Long: (Heart Block / Drugs/ Hypothyroidism)	Short: (Tachyarrhythmia, WPW, LGL, Hyperthyroidism)	
Q wave	Normal	Pathological Q wave > 25% Amplitude of R wave In which leads? I, II, III, aVL, aVF, aVR, V_1, V_2, V_3, V_4, V_5, V_6.		
QRS	Normal	Duration: < 0.1 sec.	Prolonged: RBBB, LBBB, Ventricular rhythm	
Hypertrophy / Dilatation	Left Ventricle: R (V_5) + S (V_2) > 3.5 mV Sokolow Lyon Index left vent.	Right Ventricle: R (V_2) + S (V_5) > 1.1 mV Sokolow Lyon Index right vent.	Left atrium: P Mitral (wide bifid P wave)	Right Atrium: P Pulmonal (tall peaked P wave)
ST segment	Normal	ST Elevation / ST Depression	In which leads? Antero-septal MI: V_2, V_3 Antero-lateral MI: I, aVL, V_5, V_6. Apical MI: I, aVL, V_2, V_3, V_4. Posterior wall: II, III, aVF. Right ventricle: III, aVF, aVR	

T wave	Normal: Positive in I, II, III, $V_{1,2,3,4}$	Peaked:	Flat:	Inverted:	
QTc	Normal: 0.40 - 0.44	QTc $_{Bazett}$= QT (sec) / √ RR (sec)	Long:		Short:

Diagnosis:

Recommendations:

Date:		Hospital:	Signature:

CHAPTER 9

LABORATORY TESTS

Contents

Arterial blood gases analysis	166
Complete blood count	174
Inflammation and sepsis parameters	176
Liver functions tests	178
Renal functions tests	180
Urine analysis	183
Coagulation profile	189
Pancreatic functions tests	192
Tumor markers	193
Cardiac profile tests	194
Summary and fishbone diagrams	195

ARTERIAL BLOOD GAS ANALYSIS

In this chapter we will try to simplify the results and the methods of ABG interpretations. We won't discuss any equations, theories of blood gas analysis or the buffer system of the body. Our aim is to help you to get a good grasp on the sophisticated document which called ABG.

Now we will start with simple normal values and move stepwise to interpret ABG and to reach easily to the main acid base balance disorders:

STEP 1: LOOK AT THE pH VALUE

pH value determines the state of acidity or alkalinity of the blood. Normal values are between 7.35-7.45.

Acidosis = Acidemia	< pH 7.35-7.45 <	Alkalosis = Alkalemia

After we decide, whether the Patient's blood sample is normal, academic or alkalemic, then we will search for the cause of the pathological change.

STEP 2: LOOK AT PaCO$_2$ AND HCO$_3^-$

The Lung (respiration) is responsible for PaCO$_2$ level control, and ofcourse when CO$_2$ dissolve in water (plasma), it forms Carbonic acid which is **acid. This is determined by the PaCO2 value (normal value: 40 mmHg)**

The Kidney –and other metabolic factors- are responsible for HCO$_3^-$ level control, which is **alkali. This is determined directly by the HCO3- value (normal value: 24 mEq/L)**

Simply we can now determine the initial cause of acid-base disturbance:

	Respiratory Acidosis	Metabolic Acidosis	Normal		Respiratory Alkalosis	Metabolic Alkalosis
pH State	Acidosis = Acidemia		pH 7.35-7.45		Alkalosis = Alkalemia	
Initial Change (Diagnosis)	PaCO$_2$ > 40 mmHg	HCO$_3^-$ < 24 q/L	PaCO$_2$: HCO$_3^-$: mmHg mEq/L	40 24	PaCO$_2$ < 40 mmHg	HCO$_3^-$ >24 mEq/L

Step 3: look at the Compensation = Defense mechanism of the body against pH changes.

Successful compensation aims at correcting pH changes. Partial compensation means that the body is moving in the right direction, but the pH value is not yet fully corrected. On the other hand, absent of compensatory values means failure of the compensatory mechanism to correct pH that will keep heading to a lethal value.

Normally when acidosis occurs, the body tries to react by either increasing alkalis or wash out acids from the blood –to neutralize acidosis, and vice versa in Alkalosis.

This compensation has 3 phases:

- Rapid chemical buffering e.g. HCO_3^-, Hemoglobin, intracellular protein, ammonia and phosphate.

- Intermediate respiratory compensation in the form of hypo- or hyper-ventilation which aim to change the blood levels of $PaCO_2$.

- Slow effective renal buffering by control of HCO_3^- resorption and H^+ excretion, Ammonia resorption and other titratable acids.

	Respiratory Acidosis	Metabolic Acidosis	Normal	Respiratory Alkalosis	Metabolic Alkalosis
pH State	Acidosis = Acidemia		pH 7.35-7.45	Alkalosis = Alkalemia	
Initial Change (Diagnosis)	$PaCO_2$ > 40 mmHg	HCO_3^- < 24 mEq/L	$PaCO_2$: 40 mmHg	$PaCO_2$ < 40 mmHg	HCO_3^- >24 mEq/L
Compensatory Chang	↑HCO_3^-	↓$PaCO_2$	HCO_3^- :24 mEq/L	↓HCO_3^-	↑$PaCO_2$

Congratulations!!

Now you Know the exact pathology (Acidosis or Alkalosis) the major cause of it (Respiratory or Metabolic) and the main compensatory changes using only 3 values.

ACID BASE BALANCE DISORDERS

ACIDOSIS:

Clinical effects of sever acidosis (pH<7.2):

- Sever myocardial depression and decreased cardiac output.
- Vasodilatation, hypotension and tissues hypoperfusion.
- Tissues hypoxia.
- Decrease in the vascular response for the intrinsic and extrinsic inotropes/vasoactive materials (e.g. Adrenaline and nor-adrenalin)
- Central nervous system depression esp. in cases of respiratory acidosis.
- Sever hyperkalemia (due to H+ uptake intracellular in exchange with K+)

> Sever acidosis causes sever hyperkalemia and correction of acidosis may causes sever hypokalemia.

RESPIRATORY ACIDOSIS:

Acute respiratory acidosis:

PH<7.35, PaCO2 > 40 mmHg, HCO3⁻ ≤24 mEq/l. (there is no time for renal compensation and HCO_3^- production)

Cause:

- Airway obstruction: aspiration, polytrauma, tumors, epiglottitis
- Lung problem: cardiogenic pulmonary edema, non-cardiogenic pulmonary edema e.g. burns or pneumonia, acute severe asthma.
- Pleura: pleural effusion, pneumothorax.
- Chest wall and diaphragmatic problem: obesity, flail chest.
- Muscular and neural problem: myopathy, neuropathy.
- Central nervous system: Drug induced (e.g. opioids toxicity), trauma, coma.

Chronic respiratory acidosis:

PH≤7.35, PaCO2 > 40 mmHg, HCO3⁻ >24 mEq/l. (there is enough time for renal compensation and HCO_3^- production)

Causes:

- Chronic obstructive pulmonary disease
- Chronic restrictive pulmonary diseases (obesity, lung fibrosis, restrictive pleurisy and kyphoscoliosis)

Management of respiratory acidosis:

- Correction of the cause of hypoventilation (e.g. in case of opioid toxicity give naloxone, bronchodilators in case of acute bronchial asthma)

- Decrease CO_2 production (e.g. management of Thyrotoxic crises, decrease carbohydrate intake,

- Respiratory support in the form of mechanical ventilation in case of respiratory fatigue, PH<7.2 and sever hypoxemia.

- Bicarbonate infusion (NaHCO$_3$) is indicated only if PH < 7.1 and HCO$_3^-$ < 15mEq/l.

- Chronic respiratory acidosis patient (e.g. COPD) normally has chronically high level of CO_2 in blood, so the respiratory center tolerate hypercapnia and hypoxia becomes the main stimulus for the respiratory center, so he should not receive high O_2 concentration because he depends on the hypoxic drive, otherwise bradypnea occurs followed by hypercapnia and CO_2 narcosis.

- PaCO2 in chronic respiratory acidosis patient should be partially corrected, i.e. to reach the basal PaCO2 levels.

> COPD patient should not receive high O_2 concentration because he depends on the hypoxic drive.

METABOLIC ACIDOSIS:

PH < 7.35, $PaCO_2$ < 35 mmHg., HCO_3^- <24 mEq/l.

Metabolic acidosis is classified to: high anion gap metabolic acidosis and normal anion gap metabolic acidosis.

Anion Gap = the difference between major plasma cations (Na^+) and major plasma anions (Cl^- + HCO_3^-)

Normal value = Na^+ - (Cl^- + HCO_3^-) = 140 - (104 + 24) = 12 mEq/l (accepted range: 7-14 mEq/l)

Causes: (simply)

Increased free acids level in plasma:
(high anion gap metabolic acidosis due to the presence of unmeasurable acids as keto-acids or acetylsalicylic acid)
- Diabetic-keto acidosis. DKA
- Non-ketotic hyperosmolar coma. (occurs in old DM patients)
- Lactic acidosis and starvation.
- Renal failure.
- Toxicity Salicylate, ethanol and methanol.

Decreased HCO_3^- level in plasma (± increase Cl^- level):
(normal anion gap metabolic acidosis)
- GIT loss of HCO_3^- : Diarrhea and Fistula (biliary, pancreatic, or intestinal)
- Renal loss of HCO_3^- :
- Dilutional: HCO_3^- free fluid transfusion as normal saline and some types of TPN (Hyperchloremic metabolic acidosis).

Management of Diabetic-keto acidosis DKA:

Symptoms:

fatigue, polyuria, polydipsia, nausea, vomiting and abdominal pain.

Signs:
- Patients are tachycardic, tachypneic, fever and dehydrated.
- Kussmaul's respiration (rapid, deep breathing)
- Acetone breathing odor.
- altered mental status up to coma.

Laboratory investigation:
- ABG: high anion gap metabolic acidosis.
- Serum: glucose level > 300 mg/dl., +ve ketone bodies (venous not arterial).
- Urine Analysis: Ketone bodies + Glucose.

Deferential Diagnosis:
- Hyperosmolar non-kenotic coma: old patient, sever hyperglycemia, dehydrated and minimal or no keton bodies.
- Starvation.
- Alcohol ketoacidosis: excessive alcohol consumption, vomiting and serum glucose level is normal.

Management:
- Resuscitation: Fluid – Insulin – K^+.
- Serial ABG, Electrolyte and blood glucose level.
- Prophylaxis: DVT prophylaxis.
- Treatment of the cause: treat infection, regulate insulin doses.

Fluid therapy:

(correct circulatory disturbance, correction of electrolyte imbalance and wash up keton bodies)

- Fluid deficit in DKA is about 50-100 ml/kg (correction needs between 12-24 hours to avoid brain edema)
- 1st. hour: 10 ml/kg NaCL 0.9% (= 1000 ml)
- 2nd. Hour: 5ml/kg NaCL 0.9% + K^+. (= 500 ml)
- 3^{ed}. Hour: 5ml/kg NaCL 0.9% + K^+. (= 500 ml)
- Then: 2.5ml/kg/h NaCL 0.9% + K^+. (= 250 ml/h in the next 16 h)

K^+ correction:

- if K^+ is more than 5 mmol/l then no replacement is needed
- if K^+ is lesser than 5 mmol/l. then add 20-40 mmol for each 1000ml NaCl.

Insulin therapy:

recent guidelines recommend fixed rate insulin infusion (FRII) at 0.1 IU/Kg/h

50 IU Human soluble insulin (Actrapid ^{tm} or Humulin S^{tm}) + 50 ml NaCl in 50 ml infusion pump. i.e. 1 IU/ml.

Eg. When the patient wight is 100 kg, he needs 10 IU/h = 10 ml/h.

Monitoring:
- A, B, C monitoring: Blood pressure, pulse, ECG and saturation. esp. in the first 6 hours.
- Blood gas, serum electrolyte, blood glucose level analysis each hour. esp. in the first 6 hours.
- Regular keton bodies analysis in venous blood.

ALKALOSIS:

Clinical effects of alkalosis:

Hypokalemia, decrease the plasma concentration of ionized calcium (muscle cramps), coronary vasso-spasm and decrease cerebral blood flow.

RESPIRATORY ALKALOSIS
(hyperventilation leads to decreased $PaCO_2$)

- Central causes: anxiety, psychosis, pain, salicylates toxicity, progesterone during pregnancy, analeptics, fever and sepsis.
- Peripheral causes: hypoxia, pneumonia, high altitude, heart failure, pulmonary edema and anemia.
- Iatrogenic: ventilator induced or Ambu bag induced (so it is not recommended to transport a head trauma patient without mechanical ventilator, because nearly all the patient ventilated with Ambu bag develop respiratory alkalosis which leads to decrease cerebral blood flow and further increase the brain insult).

METABOLIC ALKALOSIS
(due to excessive acids loss or excess alkalis intake)

- GIT: excessive vomiting, gastric drainage.
- Excessive diuresis.
- Endocrine causes: Hyperaldosteronism, Cushing syndrome.
- Excessive blood transfusion (due to excess citrate intake).

Management of alkalosis:

- Treatment of the cause.
- Manage the accompanying electrolyte disturbance (hypokalaemia and hypocalcaemia).

COMPLETE BLOOD COUNT

| Test | Causes of pathological findings | |
Normal findings	Increased	Decreased

Red blood cells (RBC)
4.1 – 5.6 X10^6/μL
Hemoglobin (Hb)
12.5 – 17 g/dL
	Polycythemia Vera
	
	Dehydration
	Lung disease, smoking, emphysema (chronic hypoxia)
	Polycythemia Vera
		Acute bleeding
		Bone marrow depression
		Acute or chronic bleeding,
		Bone marrow depression,
		Anemia:
		    Nutritional deficiency
		    (Iron, B12, Folate)
		    Chronic renal disease / renal anemia
		    Hemolytic anemia (sickle cell / thalassemia)

Hematocrit (Hct) 36 – 50 %	Dehydration	Microcytic anemia (Iron deficiency)
Mean corpuscular volume (MCV) 80 - 98 fL	Macrocytic anemia (B12 deficiency)	Microcytic anemia (Iron deficiency)
Mean corpuscular hemoglobin (MCH) 27 – 34 pg	Hyperchromic anemia (B12 deficiency)	Hypochromic anemia (Iron deficiency)
Mean corpuscular hemoglobin concentration (MCHC) 32 – 36 g/dL	Spherocytosis	Hypochromic anemia (Iron deficiency)
Platelets (Plt) 140 – 450 X10^3/μL	Malignancy Iron deficiency Essential thrombocytosis Postsplenectomy	Viral infection Sepsis Autoimmune thrombocytopenia Leukemia Liver cirrhosis Bone marrow depression Disseminated intravascular coagulopathy DIC
White blood cells (WBC) 4 – 11 X10^3/μL	Infection Inflammation Leukemia Severe stress Steroids	Bone marrow depression Autoimmune diseases Sepsis (overwhelming infection)

Neutrophils (Nx) 40 – 74 %	Acute bacterial infection
Lymphocytes (Lx) 14 – 46 %	Chronic infection
Monocytes (Mx) 4 – 13 %	Viral infection
Eosinophils (Ex) 0 – 7 %	Allergic reaction Parasitic infection
Basophils (Bx) 0 – 3 %	Allergic reaction Oral contraceptives

THE FISHBONE DIAGRAM

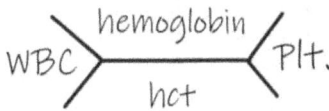

SOME COMMON DISEASES

acute bleeding

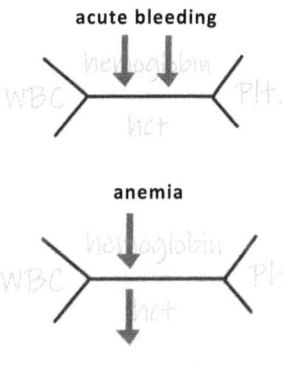

Acute bleeding: hemoglobin falls dramatically while Hematocrit remains within normal range.

Anemia: both hemoglobin and hematocrit decrease gradually. This is a good rule to evaluate initial low hemoglobin. If it is accompanied with low Hct. It is more likely to be due to anemia more than due to acute bleeding.

anemia

Pancytopenia

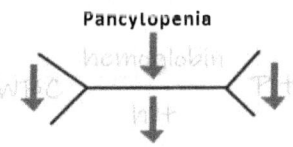

Sepsis

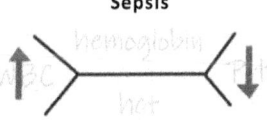

INFLAMMATION AND SEPSIS PARAMETERS

Test Normal findings	Pathological findings in infection and sepsis
White blood cells (WBC) 4 – 11 X103 /μL	Increases. 　Unspecific marker for acute inflammation. 　Deferential count for more specific determination of the cause. May decrease in severe sepsis.
C-reactive protein (CRP) < 0.5 mg/dL	Increases as follows 　✓　>0,5–<5 mg/dL: mild inflammation. 　✓　>5–<20 mg/dL: active bacterial infection. 　✓　>20 mg/dL: severe infection. Other causes of marked increase of CRP: 　Crohn's disease, neoplasia, trauma, necrosis (Myocardial infarction), Abscess and connective tissue disease (except SLE). It increases within few hours and returns to normal within 48-72 hours.
Procalcitonin (PCT) < 0.5 ng/mL	Increases as follows 　✓　>0.5–<2.0 ng/mL: moderate risk of bacterial infection. 　✓　>2.0–<10 ng/mL: high risk of bacterial infection. 　✓　>10 ng/mL: Septic shock with impending Multiple organ failure (MOF) currently the most specific parameter.
Erythrocyte sedimentation rate (ESR) < 15 ml after the first hour	Increases. 　Highly non-specific, rarely used now. 　It increases within 24 to 48 hours after the onset of acute inflammation and decreases slowly as inflammation resolves.
	Severe sepsis to septic shock
Platelets (Plt) 140 – 450 X10³ /μL	Decreases 　An early indication of septic shock
Lactate <2 mmol/L	Increases 　A value more than 1.5 times the normal value is considered significant. 　It indicates hypoxia on the cellular level due to microcirculation insufficiency.

	It leads to metabolic acidosis.
ABG	Decreases
pH 7.35-7.45	Metabolic acidosis due to tissue hypoxia (see. Lactate above).
Liver functions	Impaired liver functions as a part of Multiple organ failure (MOF).
Renal functions	Impaired renal functions as a part of Multiple organ failure (MOF).
D-Dimer	Increases
< 0.5 mg/L	Along with the thrombocytopenia can indicate the occurrence of disseminated intervascular coagulopathy (DIC) as a part of Multiple organ failure (MOF).

LIVER FUNCTIONS TESTS

Test Normal findings	Pathological findings in impaired liver functions
Alanine Aminotransferase (ALT) **Serum Glutamate Pyruvate Transferase (SGPT)** **< 40 U/L** **Aspartate Aminotransferase (AST)** **Serum Glutamate Oxaloacetate Transferase (SGOT)** **< 40 U/L**	Increases in acute liver injury ✓ Levels around few hundreds indicate mild acute hepatitis. ✓ Levels more than 1000 U/L indicate severe (fulminant) acute hepatitis. (usually ischemic, autoimmune or toxic hepatitis). ALT is more specific than AST. Increase or decrease doesn't reflect the condition of the liver function or evaluation of the level of compensation in chronic lever cell failure.
Gamma Glutamyle Transpeptidase (GGT) **< 50 U/L**	Increases in jaundice (obstructive or hepatic). More specific than ALP. False positive in chronic alcohol abuse.
Alkaline Phosphatase (alk. P) **30 – 120 U/L**	Increases in jaundice (obstructive or hepatic). Not specific Increases in other condition such as: pregnancy, increased osteoplastic activity (such as growth, fracture healing or bone metastasis).
Serum total Bilirubin (bil) **< 1.2 mg/dL** **Serum direct Bilirubin (d. bil)** **< 0.3 mg/dL**	Increases in cases of jaundice or cholestasis. The cause of jaundice can be determined according to the fraction of the direct bilirubin as follows. ✓ Normally it is about 25% of the total bilirubin. ✓ Hemolytic and hepatocellular jaundice the ratio remains at 25%. ✓ In obstructive jaundice the ratio increase more than 50%.
International Normalized Ratio (INR) **0.85 – 1.15**	Increases in acute or chronic liver function impairment. The most sensitive test of liver functions as it depends on various clotting factors that are being synthesized by the liver, such as: Factors 2, 7, 9 and 10. Other causes of increased INR: Vit. K deficiency, warfarin and hemophilia. Is one of the 5 criteria of Child-Pugh Classification.

Albumin (Alb) **3.5 – 5 g/dL**	Decreases in chronic liver function impairment. The half life of Albumin is 20 days which render it useless in evaluation of acute lever cell failure. Other causes of decreased Albumin: Protein nutritional deficiency or protein loss (nephrotic syndrome). Is one of the 5 criteria of Child-Pugh Classification.
Cholinesterase (ChE) **4.6 – 11.5 KU/L**	Decreases in chronic liver cell failure due to liver cirrhosis.

THE FISHBONE DIAGRAM

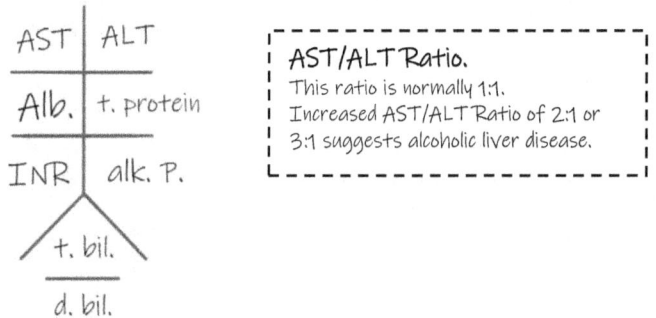

AST/ALT Ratio.
This ratio is normally 1:1.
Increased AST/ALT Ratio of 2:1 or 3:1 suggests alcoholic liver disease.

SOME COMMON DISEASES

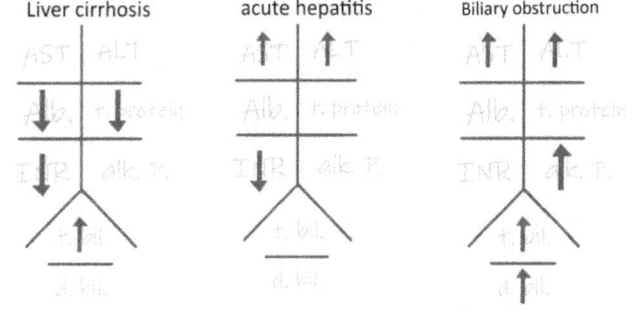

Liver cirrhosis   acute hepatitis   Biliary obstruction

RENAL FUNCTIONS TESTS

Test Normal findings	Causes of pathological findings
Serum Creatinine (Cr) Adult male: 0.6-1.2 mg/dL Adult female: 0.5-1.1 mg/dL	Parameter for the glomerular filtration rate **Increases** Impaired kidney function. Urinary tract obstruction. Muscle diseases Heart failure. Shock. **Decreases** Age extremities. Protein malnutrition. Muscle atrophy.
Urine Creatinine level Adult male: 14-26 mg/kg/24 hrs. Adult female: 11-20 mg/kg/24 hrs.	Parameter for the glomerular filtration rate, used mainly in combination with serum creatinine to calculate the glomerular filtration rate (GFR) and creatinine clearance.
Creatinine clearance Adult male: 85-125 ml/min Adult female: 75-115 ml/min.	Calculated from this formula: GFR Urine creatinine X Urine Vol. (24h) / serum creatinine X (24h) X (60min)
Glomerular filtration rate (GFR) >90 mL/min/1.73 m2	Staging of Chronic Kidney diseases (CKD) according to GFR: 0) Normal kidney function – GFR above 90 mL/min/1.73 m2 without proteinuria. 1) CKD1 – GFR above 90 mL/min/1.73 m2 with evidence of kidney damage 2) CKD2 (mild) – GFR of 60 to 89 mL/min/1.73 m2 with evidence of kidney damage 3) CKD3 (moderate) – GFR of 30 to 59 mL/min/1.73 m2 4) CKD4 (severe) – GFR of 15 to 29 mL/min/1.73 m2 5) CKD5 kidney failure – GFR less than 15 mL/min/1.73 m2
Blood-urea nitrogen (BUN) Adult: 8-21 mg/dL	Parameter of glomerular function and urea excretion. **Increases** *Renal causes:* -Acute renal failure. -Decreased renal perfusion. -Chronic glomerulonephritis. **Decreases** -Overhydration. -Hepatic disease. -Pregnancy.

-Hypovolemia.
-Nephrotoxic agents.
-Diabetes (Diabetic nephropathy)
Cardiac causes:
-Congestive heart failure.
-Shock.
-Renal Hypoperfusion.
-Ketoacidosis.
Protein Metabolism:
-Starvation/muscle wasting.
-Excessive protein intake or Protein catabolism.
-GI bleeding.
-Neoplasms.
-Tumor lysis syndrome.

-Syndrome of inappropriate anti-diuretic secretion (SIADH)
-malnutrition.
-Anabolic steroid use.
-Malabsorption syndromes.

Urea: Creatinine Ratio and BUN: Creatinine Ratio:	These correlations are used to differentiate between renal, prerenal and postrenal failure.

	Pre-renal failure	Normal or Post-renal failure	renal failure
Urea: Creatinine Ratio	>100:1	100-40:1	<40:1
BUN: Creatinine Ratio:	>20:1	20-10:1	<10:1

Serum osmolality Adult: 275-295 mosmol/kg	Evaluates hyponatremia

Increases	Decreases
Diabetes insipidus.	ADH over secretion.
Hyperglycemia.	Addison's disease.
Uremia.	Paraneoplastic syndrome (oat
Hypernatremia.	cell carcinoma).
Stroke or head trauma resulting in decreased ADH secretion.	Overhydration. Hyponatremia.
Dehydration.	Hypothyroidism.

Urine Osmolality Random specimen: 50 to 1200 mosm/kg. 12 to 14 hour fluid restriction: Greater than 850 mosmol/kg.	Evaluates body hydration.

Increases	Decreases
-Hypovolemia,	Diabetes insipidus, polydipsia
-Syndrome of inappropriate ADH secretion (SIADH).	exercise starvation.

	- Drugs: metolazone, vincristine, carbamazepine, chlorpropamide, anesthetic agents, cyclophosphamide,	Drugs: Tolazamide, Glyburide, Lithium, acetohexamide, Demeclocycline
Serum uric acid (UA) **Adult male: 4.4-7.6 mg/dL** **Adult female: 2.3-6.6 mg/dL**	**Increases with** Gout Starvation Renal failure Tumors Tumor lysis syndrome Chronic lead toxicity Diabetes Polycystic kidney disease	
Serum Sodium level (Na) **135-145 mEq/L**	**Hypernatremia** Dehydration due to excessive water loss or restricted water intake.	**Hyponatremia** Liver cirrhosis. Congestive heart failure. Nephrotic syndrome. Excessive drinking of fluids. ADH over secretion. Addison's disease. Hypothyroidism.
Potassium (K) **3.5 - 5.0 mEq/L**	**Hyperkalemia** Renal failure. Hypoaldosteronism. Rhabdomyolysis. Potassium-sparing diuretics (Spironolactone).	**Hypokalemia** Diarrhea. Medications like furosemide and steroids. Dialysis Diabetes insipidus. Hyperaldosteronism. Hypomagnesemia. Not enough intake in the diet.

THE FISHBONE DIAGRAM

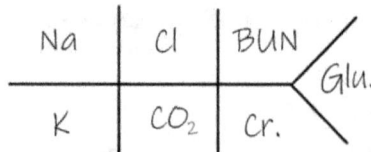

Urine Analysis

Test Normal findings	Causes of pathological findings	
A) Physical Analysis of Urin:		
1- Smell: Normally urinoid	Fruity or sweet smell: diabetic ketoacidosis Fecal smell: gastrointestinal-bladder fistula	
2- Colour: Normally yellow or amber	bright yellow: Vitamin tablets, bilirubin. Red urine: blood, hemoglobin, rifampicin. dark brown: Iron supplements, prophobilin, urobilin, levodopa, methyldopa (Aldomet) Green or blue Pseudomonal UTI, biliverdin, Amitriptyline, indigo carmine, IV cimetidine, IV promethazine or methylene blue. Milky urine may contain fat, cystine crystals, and pus cells or amorphous phosphates	
3- Transparancy: Normally urin is transparant	Turbid or cloudy: infection, pus, blood cells or fungal infection. foamy urine: glucose, bile pigment, albumin or other protein	
4- PH Urine is normally acidic 4.5 - 7.5	Low pH (acidic): high protein diet metabolic or respiratory acidosis diabetic ketoacidosis. Diarrhoea starvation	High pH (alkaline): Low carbohydrate diet. certain vegetables, citrus fruits, and milk products. Respiratory or metabolic alkalosis Urinary tract infection (bacteria convert urea → ammonia, which is highly alkaline)
5- Specific Gravity: Normally around 1.010	Low Spicific Gravity: (dilution) Excessive fluid intake Diuritics Acute renal failure, acute tubular necrosis (Diuresis phase). Acute glomerulonephritis. pyelonephritis. Diabetes insipidus.	High Specific Gravity:(concentration) Dehydration. Heart failure. Liver failure. vomiting or diarrhea DM (high glucose concentration)

6- **Volume:** Normally urine volume is between 600 – 2000 ml/24h or more than 0.5ml/kg/h	Increased (Polyuria) > 2000ml/24h e.g. Diabetic mellitus Diabetic insipidus Acromegaly Myxedema tubular necrosis	Decreased (Oliguria) < 400ml/24h or < 0.5 ml/kg/h e.g. Impaired renal perfusion Dehydration. Heart failure. Liver failure. Sepsis. vomiting or diarrhea mechanical obstruction of the urinary tract.

B) Chemical analysis of Urine

1- **Sugar (Glucose)** Normally less than 15- 20 mg/dl	Glycosuria: Urine Glucose > 15- 20 mg/dl **Physiological causes:** - After carbohydrates ingestion. - Sympathetic stimulants such as stress. - Renal Glycosuria: due to congenital lowered renal threshold. - Pregnancy may be associated with physiological glycosuria. **Pathological Glycosuria:** - Diabetes mellitus when blood glucose level exceeds 170 - 180 mg/dl (renal threshold), glucose appears in urine - Hyperthyroidism - Hyperadrenalism - Hyperpitutarism
2- **Ketone Bodies:** (acetone, acetoacetate, and β –hydroxybutyrate) Normally: not detectable in the blood or urine.	**Ketonuria:** - starvation. - diabetes mellitus (DKA). - prolonged vomiting. - severe diarrhea. - anesthesia. - severe liver damage. - high fat intake and/or low carbohydrate diet.
3- **Protein:** Normally: not or minimal detectable in the blood or urine.	**Causes of Proteinuria:** 1. Increased permeability of the glomerulus: e.g. glomerular membrane is damaged 2. decreased tubular reabsorption of the little amount of protein which is filtrated throughout the glomeruli (with lower molecular weight)
- **Albumin.**	Physical Exercise. **1+** = (50 mg/dL). Emotional Stress. **2+** = (200 mg/dL). Infections. **3+** = (500 mg/dL).

		Glomerulonephritis. **4+** = (1000mg/dL or more)
		Nephrotic Syndrom.
		Newborns.
		Pregnancy.
-	Globulins	Glomerulonephritis.
		Tubular Dysfunction
-	Bence Jones protein	Multiple Myeloma
		Leukemia
-	Hemoglobin	Hematuria.
		Hemoglobinuria.

4- Bilirubin:
Normally: up to 0.02 mg/dl

- Early sign of liver cell disease (hepatocellular disease)
- Obstruction of the bile flow from the liver (Obstructive or post - hepatic jaundice).

Bilirubin is red-brown when voided, and turns to the green color on standing (Bilirubin → Biliverdin).

5- Urobilinogen:
Normally: trace amount

Increased Urobilinogen:
- Hemolytic jaundice
- Impaired liver function is impaired

6- Hemoglobin

Hemoglobinuria occurs due to severe intravascular hemolysis:

- Hemolytic anemia:
    - Glucose - 6- phosphate dehydrogenase (G6PD) deficiency.
    - Sickle cell disease.
    - Drug induced.
    - Snake bites.
    - Incompatible blood transfusion.
- Severe infectious disease: Yellow Fever, Small Pox and Typhoid Fever.
- Malaria.
- Sever septicaemia.
- Incompatible blood transfusion.
- Poisonings with strong acids or mushrooms
- Sever-burns.
- Renal infarction.

7- Serum Calcium

24-hour Urine collection and Ca^{++} level determination test is ordered to determine the function of the parathyroid gland.

Hyperparathyroidism: due to increased secretion of parathyroid hormones and an increased excretion of urinary calcium.

Hypoparathyroidism: the urinary calcium is decreased.

False positive:	False negatives
- High sodium and magnesium intake.	- Increased dietary phosphates.

		- Excess milk intake. - Alkaline urine. - After high dietary Ca^{++} intake. - Drugs.
8-	Nitrite	The presence of nitrite is indication of urinary tract infection.
9-	Melanin	The presence of Melanin is indication of malignant melanoma esp. when accompined with hepatic metastasis.
10-	Vanillylmandelic acid (VMA)	The presence of Vanillylmandelic acid is indication of presence of neuroendocrine tumors, such as neuroblastomas and pheochromocytomas.

C)	Microscopic Urine Examination:
	a- Cells:

1-	Red blood cells RBC's
	Normally less than 5 RBC's / HPF[11].
		Causes:
		1- Inflammatory and traumatic causes:
		       Renal stone
		       Acute and chronic glomerulonephritis
		       Trauma of the kidney
		       Cystitis.
		       Prostatitis.
		2- Tumours:
		       Renal malignancies.
		       Urinary bladder carcinome.
		       Prostatic tumours.
		3- Haemorrhagic tendencies:
		       Haemphilia.
		       Liver failure.
		       Anticoagulants.
		       Malignant hypertension.
		4- Rare conditions:
		       TB urinary tract, Schistosoma
		5- Misinterpretation:
		       Vaginal bleeding.
		6- Transient, temporarily hematuria after exercise.

2-	Leukocytes WBC's	**Causes:** - Urinary tract infection. - Renal tubuler diseases.

---

[11] HPF: high power field

Normally less than 5 WBC 's / HPF.	- Bladder tumor. - Cystitis. - Prostatitis.
3- Epithelial cells: Normally less than 3 cells / HPF.	Acute tubular damage. Tubular necrosis. Acute glomerulonephritis Silicate over dose
4- Spermatozoa	Retrograde ejaculation (polyneuropathy)

b- Casts:

1- Hyaline Casts: Normally 0-2/HPF	Causes: Hyaline casts occurs due to increased protein leak through the glomerular membrane. - Nephritis. - Chronic renal disease. - Congestive heart failure. - Diabetic nephropathy. - Fever. - Postural orthostatic strain. - Emotional stress. - Exercise.
2- Granular Casts:	Causes: - Acute tubular necrosis - Granulonephritis - Pyelonephrites - Lead poisoning - exercise
3- Waxy Casts	Causes: - Indicator of progressive renal damage: - Chronic renal disease. - Tubular degeneration.
4- Fatty Casts	Causes: - Important sign of nephritic syndrome. - Chronic renal disease. - Degeneration of renal tubules.
5- Cellular Casts	- Red cell cast → acute glomerulonephritis cases. - White blood cell casts → pyelonephritis. - Epithelial casts → tubular degeneration.

c- Parasites:

1- Trichomonas Vaginalis	- Trichomonas Vaginaitis - Urinary tract infection.
2- Wuchereria Bancroftie	Tissue nematode that invades lymph vessels causing lymphedema (elephantiasis) in lower limb. It may be accompanied with chyluria (lymph in urine)
3- Schistosoma Haematobium	- Schistosomiasis or Bilharsiasis

d-	**Yeast cells**	Fungal infection of the urinary tract occurs in immune suppressed patient:
		- Diabetic mellitus.
		- Intensive antibiotic therapy.
		- Immunosuppressive therapy
		Vaginal candidiasis.

	e-	**Crystals:**	
1-	**Amorphous Urates**	Normal finding
2-	**Uric Acid Crystals**	Normal finding (little amount)
		Increased in :
		- Gout
		- Celluller distruction (Malignancies +/- Chemotherapy)
3-	**Cystine Crystals**	Acute pyelonephritis
		Willson's disease
4-	**Cholesterol**	Chylurea
		Advanced hyperlipidemia.
5-	**Calcium Oxalate Crystal**	- Calcium and oxalate rich foods: milk, tomatoes, asparagus, mango, strawberry and orange
		- Dehydration.
		- Chronic renal disease:
		- Urinary stones.
6-	**Amorphous Phosphates**	Indicates that the urine is alkaline.
7-	**Calcium Phosphates**	Cystitis

COAGULATION PROFILE

Test Normal findings	Causes of pathological findings	
Platelets (Plt) 140 – 450 X103 /µL	**Increases** Malignancy Iron deficiency Essential thrombocytosis Postsplenectomy	**Decreases** Viral infection Sepsis Autoimmune thrombocytopenia Leukemia Liver cirrhosis Bone marrow depression Disseminated intravascular coagulopathy DIC
International Normalized Ratio (INR) 0.85 – 1.15 Prothrombin Time (PT) 12 – 13 seconds Prothrombin Ratio (Quick) 70 – 130 %	They increase in bleeding tendency (except Prothrombin ration which decreases). They asses the functions of the extrinsic and the common pathways. **Causes of related bleeding tendency:** Acute or chronic liver insult or liver function deterioration. Warfarin therapy. Vit. K deficiency Hemophilia Sepsis und DIC	
Activated partial thromboplastin time (aPTT) 26 – 36 seconds	Increases in bleeding tendency. assesses the functions of the intrinsic and the common pathways. **Causes of related bleeding tendency:** Heparin therapy Von Willebrand's disease Factors VIII, IX, XI and XII deficiency Hemophilia Sepsis und DIC	
Plasma Thrombin Time (PTT) 17 – 24 seconds	Increases in bleeding tendency. assesses the conversion of fibrinogen to fibrin. **Causes of related bleeding tendency:** Fibrinogen deficiency.	
D-Dimer	Increases in abnormal thrombosis.	

< 0.5 mg/L	It is an end product of fibrin degradation. **Causes of increased D-Dimer:** DVT Pulmonary embolism After surgery or trauma Chronic inflammation D-Dimer is more of a good negative in pulmonary embolism and DVT than a diagnostic test.

FACTOR	NAME
I	Fibrinogen
II	Prothrombin
III	Tissue factor or thromboplastin
IV	Calcium
V	Proaccelerin (Labile factor)
VII	Proconvertin (Stable factor)
VIII	Antihaemophilic factor A
IX	Antihaemophilic factor B
X	Stuart-Prower factor
XI	Plasma thromboplastin antecedent, Haemophilia C
XII	Hageman factor
XIII	Fibrin stabilising factor

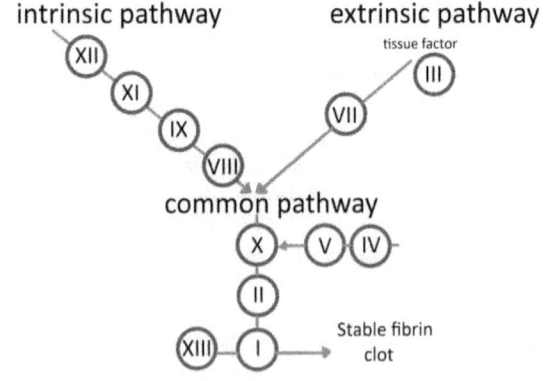

THE FISHBONE DIAGRAM

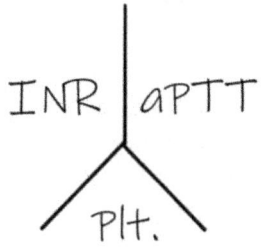

INR | aPTT
Plt.

SOME COMMON DISEASES

Warfarin therapy
liver cirrhosis

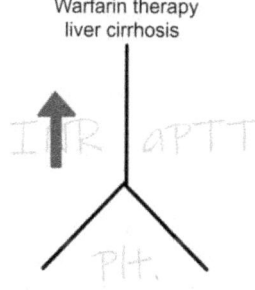

thrombocytopenia

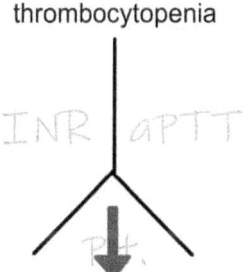

DIC

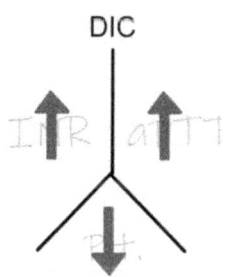

Hemophilia
heparin therapy

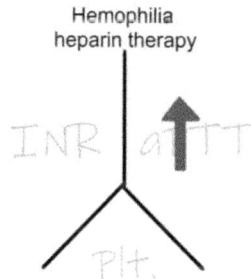

PANCREATIC FUNCTIONS[12]

Test Normal findings	Causes of pathological findings	

Serum Amylase
<100 U/L
Serum Lipase
<60 U/L
	Both increase in acute pancreatitis.
	    A 3-fold increase is usually clinically significant.
	    Lipase is specific to pancreatic insult, while amylase can also increase in salivary glands inflammation (parotidis).
	Both may increase with renal failure.
	    due to reduced renal elimination.
	Both may decrease in chronic pancreatitis
	    due to reduced pancreatic exocrine functions.	

	Prediabetes (Glucose Intolerance)	Diabetes
Fasting glucose 55 – 100 mg/dL	100–125 mg/dL	≥126 mg/dL
Postprandial glucose (120 minutes) <140 mg/dL	140–199 mg/dL	≥200 mg/dL
Random glucose <140 mg/dL		≥200 mg/dL
Glycated hemoglobin (HbA$_{1c}$) 4 – 6 %	5.7–6.4%	≥6.5%

---

[12] Reference numbers for diagnosis of diabetes and prediabetes are based on the American Diabetes Association. http://www.diabetes.org/diabetes-basics/diagnosis/

TUMOR MARKERS

Test	Acronym	Normal range	Unit	Primary Tumor Type
Carcinoembryonic antigen	CEA	< 5	ng/mL	Colorectal carcinoma
Alfa feto protein	AFP	< 20	ng/mL	Hepatocellular carcinoma Non-seminiferous testicular tumors
Beta human chorionic gonadotropin	B-hCG	< 3	mIU/mL	choriocarcinoma
Calcitonin		2-10 (female) 2-48 (male)	ng/L	Medullary thyroid carcinoma
Metanephrines		12-60	Pg/mL	Pheochromocytoma
Cancer Antigen	CA 15-3	< 30	U/mL	Breast Cancer
	CA 19-9	37-40	U/mL	Pancreatic and Gastric carcinoma
	CA 72-4	< 4	U/mL	Gastric carcinoma
	CA 125	46	U/mL	Ovarian Carcinoma
Prostate specific antigen	PSA	< 4	ng/mL	Prostate Carcinoma

CARDIAC PROFILE TESTS

Coronary Artery Disease assessment

Group I	1.	Blood Glucose level→ Hyperglycemia (DM).
	2.	Blood Urea Level→ Hyperuricemia (Renal insufficiency).
Cardiac risk	3.	Serum Electrolytes→ Hyperkalemia (Renal insufficiency).
assessment	4.	Serum creatinine → Elevated serum creatinine (Renal insufficiency).
Group II	1-	Serum HDL. > 1.0 mmol/l = 60mg/dl.
	2-	Serum LDL < 3.0 mmol/l = 100mg/dl.
Cardiac risk	3-	Serum Total Cholesterol < 5.0 mmol/l = 200mg/dl.
evaluation tests	4-	Serum Triglyceride < 2.0 mmol/l = 150 mg/dl.
	5-	Serum non-HDL Cholesterol < 3.9 mmol/l.
	6-	Homocysteine: Predisposing factor for coronary artery disease.
	7-	Apo lipoproteins: Assess prognostic values of lipid lowering drug therapy and risk of CAD, Apoprotein A, B, B100: 100-120 mg/dl.
Group III	1-	Serum Creatine Phospho-Kinase (CPK).
	2-	Serum Glutamate Oxaloacetate Transferase (SGPT).
Cardiac injury	3-	Serum Lactate Dehydrogenase (LDH).
evaluation tests	4-	Serum Hydro Butyrate Dehydrogenase (SHBD).
	5-	Myoglobin.
	6-	CK-MB.
	7-	Troponin I/T.

Cardiac Marker	Increases	Peak	Return to Baseline	Comments
A- Second Generation: (biomarkers)				
Myoglobin	1–4 h	4–12 h	24–36 h	Early but not cardiac-specific marker
Troponin I	4–9 h	12–24 h	7–14 days	Highly specific
Troponin T	4–9 h	12–24 h	7–14 days	Highly specific
B- First Generation: (enzymes)				
Total CK	3-12 h	24 h	48–72 h	Non-specific
CK-MB	3–12 h	24 h	48–72 h	Relative specific
LDH 1, 2	6-12 h	72 h	7-14 days	Less specific, late diagnosis
SGOT	6-12 h	24-48 h	4-6 days	Less specific

SUMMARY

THE FISHBONE DIAGRAMS

The fishbone diagram is a good way to summarize the laboratory tests results of your patient.

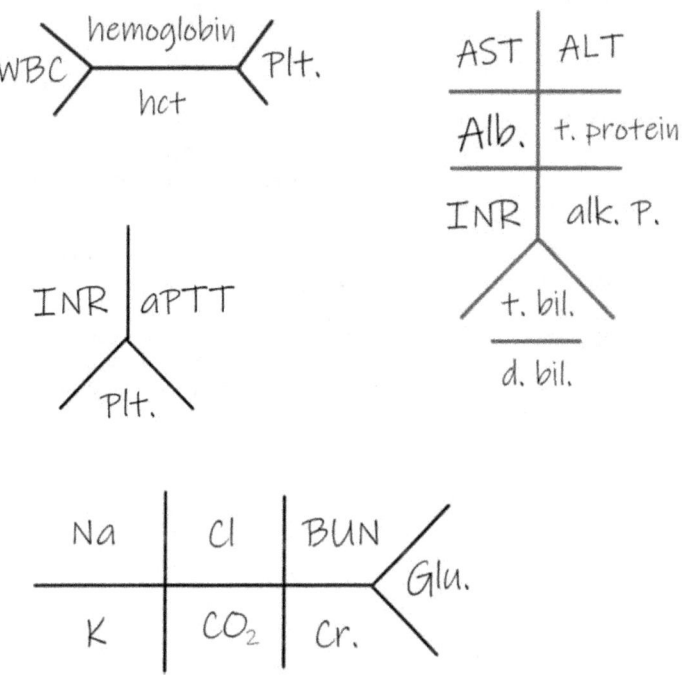

AUTHORS' BIOGRAPHY

Mina Azer got his Master's degree in surgery in 2013. He has a great passion for science yielded in his current research and publications. Between 2004 and 2016 he shared in more than 70 different training delivered to more than 2000 trainees about various topics such as: reproductive health, surgical skills, and medical research. He worked at the Gastroenterology Surgical Center in Mansoura University, Egypt and at the Egyptian Liver Research Institute and Hospital. He is currently working at the Ubbo-Emmius Klinik in Norden, Germany.

Romany Azer got his Master's Degree and completed a residency in anesthesia, surgical Intensive care and pain medicine in 2009 in the educational Zagazig university hospitals, then he worked as anesthetist and assistant lecturer for anesthesia in the Faculty of medicine, Zagazig university in Egypt. Dr. Azer has shared in multiple research works and teaching procedures for the medical students (the science of anesthesia, intensive care, emergency medicine and pain medicine), in 2015 he got his Doctor title in anesthesia, surgical intensive care pain medicine, and then worked as a Lecturer in the same university, he shared as lecturer and trainer in multiple national and international anesthesia and pain congresses. In 2016 he started to work in Germany as anesthetist in Ubbo-Emmius Hospital group (Norden-Aurich), he started in 2019 as anesthetist and pain therapist at the Christliches Krankenhaus Quackenbrück- Germany - the academic educational Hospital of Oldenburg university (Germany) and the European medical school Groningen (Holland).

Dear colleague,

Did we do a good job?
Is everything OK?
Is something missing?
Did we oversee something?
Perhaps a typo?
Is something outdated?

Your opinion is most appreciated. Please don't hesitate to contact us to share your insights to help us doing a better job in the next editions. Also like our Facebook page to stay tuned for updates, posters and cheat sheets.

All the best,

Yours,

Mina Azer
Email: meena_tharwat@yahoo.co.uk

Romany Azer
Email: r.azer@ ckq-gmbh.de

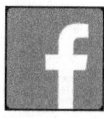

Facebook Page: A2Z in ER
https://www.facebook.com/A2ZinER